CBS Confident Pharmacy Series

Health Education and Community Pharmacy

Third Edition

for First Year Diploma in Pharmacy

(**0810**) Strictly Based on Syllabus as per ER1991

V.N. Raje M Pharm

Principal
Gourishankar Education Society's
GES College of Pharmacy (D Pharm)
Limb, Satara, Maharashtra

CBS Publishers & Distributors Pvt Ltd

New Delhi • Bengaluru • Chennai • Kochi • Kolkata • Mumbai
Hyderabad • Jharkhand • Nagpur • Patna • Pune • Uttarakhand

Disclaimer

Science and technology are constantly changing fields. New research and experience broaden the scope of information and knowledge. The author has tried his best in giving information available to him while preparing the material for this book. Although, all efforts have been made to ensure optimum accuracy of the material, yet it is quite possible some errors might have been left uncorrected. The publisher, the printer and the author will not be held responsible for any inadvertent errors or inaccuracies.

Health Education and Community Pharmacy

Third Edition

ISBN: 978-93-86478-52-8

Third Edition: 2018
Reprint: 2018, 2019, 2020, 2021 2022
First Edition: 2010
Reprint: 2011
Second Edition: 2015
Reprint: 2016

Published by Satish Kumar Jain and produced by Varun Jain for

CBS Publishers & Distributors Pvt Ltd

4819/Xi Prahlad Street, 24 Ansari Road, Daryaganj, New Delhi 110 002, India.
Ph: 011-23289259, 23266861, 23266867 Website: www.cbspd.com
Fax: 011-23243014 e-mail: delhi@cbspd.com; cbspubs@airtelmail.in.
Corporate Office: 204 FIE, Industrial Area, Patparganj, Delhi 110 092
Ph: 011-4934 4934 Fax: 011-4934 4935 e-mail: publishing@cbspd.com; publicity@cbspd.com

Branches

- **Bengaluru:** Seema House 2975, 17th Cross, K.R. Road, Banasankari 2nd Stage, Bengaluru 560 070, Karnataka
  Ph: +91-80-26771678/79 Fax: +91-80-26771680 e-mail: bangalore@cbspd.com
- **Chennai:** 7, Subbaraya Street, Shenoy Nagar, Chennai 600 030, Tamil Nadu
  Ph: +91-44-26680620, 26681266 Fax: +91-44-42032115 e-mail: chennai@cbspd.com
- **Kochi:** 42/1325, 1326 Power House Road, Opp. KSEB, Kochi 682018, Kerala
  Ph: +91-484-4059061-65 Fax: +91-484-4059065 e-mail: kochi@cbspd.com
- **Kolkata:** 6/B, Ground Floor, Rameswar Shaw Road, Kolkata-700 014, West Bengal
  Ph: +91-33-22891126, 22891127, 22891128 e-mail: kolkata@cbspd.com
- **Mumbai:** 83-C, Dr E Moses Road, Worli, Mumbai-400018, Maharashtra
  Ph: +91-22-24902340/41 Fax: +91-22-24902342 e-mail: mumbai@cbspd.com

Representatives

- **Hyderabad** 0-9885175004
- **Jharkhand** 0-9811541605
- **Nagpur** 0-9421945513
- **Patna** 0-9334159340
- **Pune** 0-9623451994
- **Uttarakhand** 0-9716462459

Printed at Mudrak, Noida, UP, India

to

my beloved family

CBS Confident Pharmacy Series

Health Education and Community Pharmacy

Third Edition

for First Year Diploma in Pharmacy

(**0810**) Strictly Based on Syllabus as per ER1991

Question–Answer Type Notes and Board Question Papers (1997 to 2017)

Salient Features

- Total Confidence and 100 percent Success in Every Examination.
- Repeatedly Asked Board Questions Indicated in Brackets.
- Chapterwise Collection of Very Important Questions.
- Written in Very Simple and Lucid Language.
- Board Question Papers 2015–2017 given at the End of Text.

CBS Titles by the same Author in

CBS Confident Pharmacy Series

First Year D Pharm

1. Pharmaceutics I, 3/e
2. Pharmaceutical Chemistry I, 3/e
3. Pharmacognosy, 3/e
4. Biochemistry and Clinical Pathology, 3/e
5. Human Anatomy and Physiology, 3/e
6. Health Education and Community Pharmacy, 3/e

Second Year D Pharm

1. Pharmaceutics II, 3/e
2. Pharmaceutical Chemistry II, 3/e
3. Pharmacology and Toxicology, 3/e
4. Pharmaceutical Jurisprudence, 3/e
5. Drug Store and Business Management, 3/e
6. Hospital and Clinical Pharmacy, 3/e

Preface to the Third Edition

The third edition of the now popular and successful book includes Board Question Papers 1997 to 2017. The book has been written to meet the requirements of students of Diploma in Pharmacy (D Pharm) in accordance with the new revised syllabus ER1991 prescribed by Pharmacy Council of India.

This book is small and humble effort has been put in for compiling necessary information on the subject. An attempt has been made to demystify and simplify the basic concepts for the students of pharmacy and to enable them get an evergreen success in MSBTE examinations.

The salient features of the present book are:

- Lucid and easy language,
- To the point answers,
- Remembering facts in the simplest way, and
- Infusing confidence in the reader to appear in the Board Examinations.

Hence the series is named

CBS Confident Pharmacy Series

I am confident that this book will be useful to both the students and the teachers of Diploma in Pharmacy as well as the candidates desiring to succeed in competitive examinations for better job opportunities in pharmacy profession such as hospital pharmacists in PHCs, civil hospitals, etc.

Raje Vijay N

Acknowledgements

I express my heartfelt thanks to Prof Madan Jagtap, Chairman, Gourishankar Education Society, Satara Maharashtra, for consistent encouragement and inspiration for writing this book.

I wish to acknowledge the prompt and efficient help given by Prof Milind Jagtap, Mr Jaywant Salunkhe, Mr Appa Rajage, Mr Nitin Mudalgikar, and Mr Shrirang Katekar of Gourishankar Education Society, Satara.

I am also thankful to Shri Satish Kumar Jain, Chairman and Managing Director, and Shri RN Mandal, General Manager, Pune Branch, CBS Publishers & Distributors Pvt Ltd, for their sustained efforts and keen interest in the publication of this book.

I wish all my beloved students to have a great success in the Board Examinations.

Raje Vijay N

Syllabus

(As per ER 1991)

Health Education and Community Pharmacy

1. Concept of health—Definition of physical health, mental health, social health, spiritual health—determinants of health, indicators of health. Concept of disease, natural history of diseases, the diseases agents, concept of prevention of diseases.
2. Nutrition and health—Classification of foods, requirements, diseases induced due to deficiency of proteins, vitamins and mineral—treatment and prevention.
3. Demography and family planning—Demography cycle, fertility, family planning, contraceptive methods, behavioral methods, natural family planning methods, chemical methods, mechanical methods, hormonal contraceptive, population problem of India.
4. First Aid—Emergency treatment in shock-snake, bite, burns, poisoning, heart disease, fractures and resuscitation methods. Elements of minor surgery and dressings.
5. Environment and health—Sources of water supply, water pollution, purification of water, health and air, noise, light—solid waste disposal and control-medical entomology, arthropod borne diseases and their control, rodents, animals and diseases.
6. Fundamental principle of microbiology—Classification of microbes, isolation, staining techniques of organisms of common diseases.
7. Communicable diseases—Causative agents, mode of transmission and prevention.
   a. Respiratory infections—Chicken pox, Measles, Influenza, Diphtheria, Whooping cough and Tuberculosis.
   b. Intestinal infections—Poliomyelitis, Hepatitis, Cholera, Typhoid, Food poisoning, Hookworm infection.
   c. Arthropod borne infections—Plague, Malaria, Filariasis.
   d. Surface infections—Rabies, Trachoma, Tetanus, Leprosy.
   e. Sexually transmitted diseases—Syphilis, Gonorrhoea, AIDS.

8. Noncommunicable diseases—Causative agents, prevention, care and control cancer, Diabetes, Blindness, Cardiovascular diseases.
9. Epidemiology—its scope, methods, uses, dynamics of disease transmission, immunity and immunization.
   Immunological products and prevention, hospital acquired infection, prevention and control. Disinfection, types of disinfection procedures, for faeces, urine, sputum, room, linen, dead-bodies, instruments.

Contents

CHAPTER 1

Concept of Health

Q 1. Define the term "health". (S. 95, 97, 98, 02, 00, 05, 06, 07; W. 97, 99, 00, 01, 02, 04, 05, 06, 08)

According to World Health Organization (WHO) the term health is defined as:

"Health is a state of complete physical, mental and social well-being and not merely an absence of disease or infirmity."

Q 2. Mention various dimensions/types/aspects of health. (S. 96, 97, 05, 06, 07, 08; W. 96, 99, 00, 01, 02, 05, 06)

The concept of health refers to many aspects or dimensions such as:

- Physical health or physical dimension.
- Mental health or mental dimension.
- Social health or social dimension.
- Spiritual health or spiritual dimension.
- Emotional health or emotional dimension.
- Vocational health or vocational dimension.

Q 3. Describe in brief about physical health. (S. 03; W. 97)

Physical Health

It is defined as "a state in which every cell and every organ is functioning at optimum capacity and in perfect harmony with the rest of the body".

- It refers to the perfect functioning of the body.
- It indicates that all body organs are structurally and functionally in a normal state and there is a perfect coordination between the organs and the systems.

- The signs of physical health in an individual are as follows:
  - A good complexion
  - Clean skin
  - Bright eyes
  - Lustrous hair
  - Not too fat
  - Good appetite
  - Sound sleep
  - Regular activity of bowel and bladder
  - Smooth and easy coordinated movements
  - Body weight, pulse rate, BP, etc. are all in normal limits
  - A sweet breath
- The physical health can be assessed by clinical examination, nutrition and biomedical and laboratory investigations.

Q 4. What is mental health? State major types of mental disorders. (S. 00, 01, 03; W. 99)

Mental Health

Mental health has been defined as "a state of balance between the individual and the surrounding world including environment and a state of harmony between oneself and others".

Types of Mental Disorders/Diseases

- *Psychosis*: It is the psychic condition which involves marked impairment of behaviour with a serious inability to think.
- *Neurosis*: This term is used to denote less severe form of psychosis.
- *Schizophrenia*: It is psychic condition characterized by disturbed thinking and emotional withdrawal from surrounding.
- *Depression*: It is a common psychiatric disorders characterized by a feeling of misery, apathy, hopelessness, ugliness, loss of appetite, insomnia, anorexia, alteration in moods and activities, etc.

Q 5. Write a note on mental health. (S. 95, 96, 99, 00, 03; W. 97, 99)

Mental Health

"It is a state of balance between the individual and the surrounding world including environment and a state of harmony between oneself and others."

- Mental health refers to mind of the individual.
- It is always said that healthy mind resides in healthy body.
- Therefore, physical and mental components of health are indivisible.

- Mental health is an ability of individual to adjust with the environment and the surrounding world.

Characteristics/Signs of Mentally Healthy Person

- He is free from internal conflicts.
- He is well adjusted with surrounding.
- He searches for identity.
- He knows himself, his needs, problems and goals.
- He has a good self-control.
- He faces problems and tries to solve them intelligently.

Q 6. Write a brief about "social health". (S. 99, 03)

Social Health

It has been defined as "a quantity and quality of an individual interpersonalities and the extent of involvement with the community.

- Man is social animal, he cannot live individually, he will have to depend on each other to fulfill his basic needs.
- Thus the social health implies harmony and integration within the individual and members of the society and the world in which they live.
- The social health considers the individual as a member of society and his health status in relation to socioeconomic conditions of the social group in which he lives.

Q 7. Write a short note on "spiritual health/holistic health".

Spiritual Health

It is concerned with spirit or soul which directs the person towards right things and keeps away from bad habits.

- Spiritual health plays a role in health and disease.
- Spiritual health refers to that part of the individual which reaches out and strives from meaning and purpose in life.
- Spiritual health may determine or influence individual's physiology and psychology.
- The body is always guided by soul, if the spiritual health is sound, the bad thinking is always controlled by inner soul.
- All religions are concerned mainly about the spiritual welfare.
- Spiritual health is the supernatural power that contributes to the health of an individual.

- Spiritual component of health is necessary to follow the rules and regulations in daily life.
- To do prayers in the morning and evening is healthy sign of spiritual health.

Q 8. Discuss various variables/determinants/factors which govern the health of an individual. (S. 96, 97, 98, 03, 04, 05, 07, 09; W. 99, 00, 02, 07, 08)

Determinants of Health

"The factors which influence the health of the individual and external environment or society where he lives are called as determinants of health."

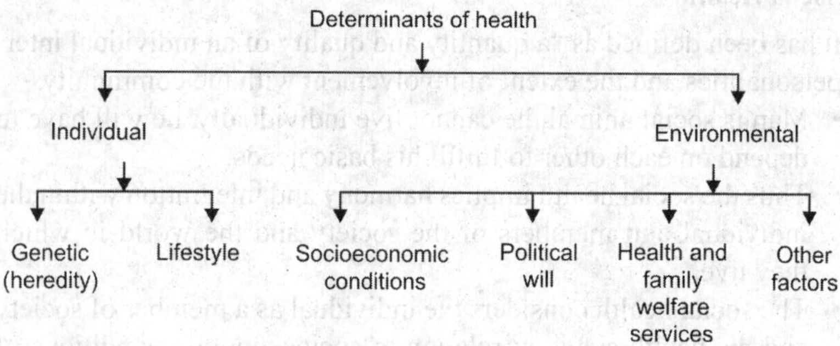

Individual

- *Genetic* (*heredity*): The state of health depends upon genetic constituent of man. Genes play a very important role in the health and development of child. Many diseases are hereditary, e.g. hemophilia and sickle cell anemia, diabetes occurs in the next generations which affect the health.
- *Lifestyle*: The lifestyle is the way people live. Lifestyle of an individual plays a great role in health. Many health problems are associated with lifestyle changes or personal habits such as smoking, alcoholism, etc. Some lifestyles can promote the health which include care of body, bathing, washing, care of teeth, hair, nail, adequate sleep, nutrition. Thus there is an association between health and lifestyle of an individual.

Environment/Surrounding Factors

- *Socioeconomic conditions*: These conditions influence human health. The economic status, purchasing power, education, occupation, family size, quality of life affect the health status of an individual in many ways.

- *Political will*: The health is also related to country's political system. A political system oriented towards social development promotes good health.

  The poor people living in slums, lacking good hygienic conditions are the targets of disease agents. The people in rural areas who do not have access to health services should be taken into consideration while framing the health policies by the political parties because it ultimately affects the health status of these communities.
- *Health and family welfare services*: It covers personal and community services for the prevention, treatment of disease and promotion of health.

  The purpose of health services is to improve health status. It includes services like immunization, safe water supply, care of pregnant woman and children, treatment of sterility, framing "small family norm", etc. For these activities "primary health centres" are good places of operation.
- *Other factors*: Other factors contributing to the health-derived policies such as employment, opportunities, education, rural developments, etc.

Q 9. What do you mean by "indicators of health"? Give the characteristics of an ideal indicator. (S. 98, 00, 01; W. 98, 02)

Indicators of Health

Health indicators are the factors used to measure the health status of community as well as to find out how far a given person is healthy.

Characteristics of an Ideal Health Indicator

- It should be valid.
- It should be reliable.
- It should be sensitive.
- It should be specific.

Q 10. Write a note on "economic cycle of disease". (S. 04; W. 02)

The health of an individual depends on the socioeconomic factors which are governed by set rules of regulations framed and accepted by the society in which he lives.

Therefore, poor economic status, poor nutrition, poor education, poor housing are major root causes of the diseases and affects health status of an individual.

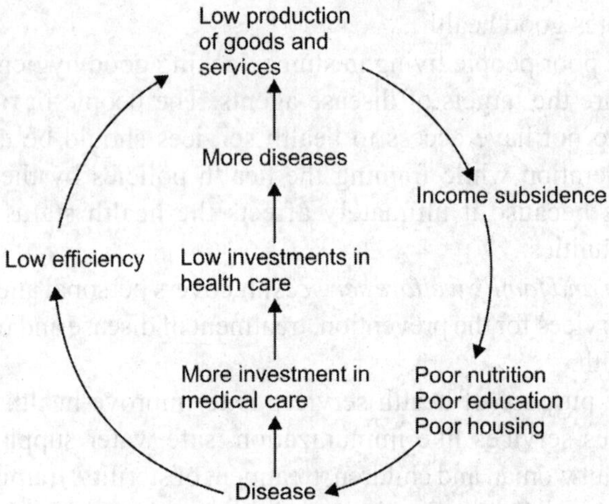

Economic cycle of disease

Q 11. Enlist various indicators of health (classify indicators of health). (S. 95, 98, 01, 08; W. 98, 02, 03, 05, 07)

Indicators of health are classified as:
- Mortality indicators.
- Morbidity indicators.
- Disability indicators.
- Nutritional status indicators.
- Health care delivery indicators.
- Utilization indicators.
- Indicators of social and mental health.
- Environmental indicators.
- Socioeconomic indicators.
- Health policy indicators.
- Quality of life indicators.
- Other indicators such as sanitation indicator.

Q 12. Write a note on mortality indicators (death rate). (S. 04; W. 98, 99, 04)

- Mortality rate means death rate.

- Mortality rate of children of any country is the direct indicator for judging the state of development of the country.
- A high mortality rate of children in a country indicates that the country is undeveloped.
- Mortality indicators may be classified as:
  i. *Crude death rate*: It is defined as number of deaths per 1000 population per year in a given community.
     – It indicates the rate at which the people are dying.
  ii. *Expectation of life*: Expectancy of life at birth is the average number of years likely to be lived by a person if current age specific mortality rates are applied.
     – If the expectation of life increases it indicates improvement in the health status and socioeconomic development.
     – To achieve expectancy of life at birth, 60 years is the target for "health for all" by 2000 AD.
  iii. *Infant mortality rate*: It is the rate of deaths under 1 year of age in a given year to total number of live birth in same year.
  iv. *Child mortality rate*: It is defined as the number of deaths at ages 1–4 years in a given year per 1000 children in that age group.
  v. *Maternal mortality rate*: It is the proportion of total deaths occurring in the women of reproductive age.

Q 13. What do you mean by morbidity indicators? (W. 98, 99)

Morbidity indicators give information regarding the disease situations in the community.

- The morbidity rate (disease rate) is the number of cases of a disease found to occur in a stated number of population.
- Morbidity indicators are used for assessing ill-health in the community which is not judged by mortality indicators.
- Morbidity indicators include:
  i. Incidence and prevalence rate.
  ii. Epidemiological studies.
  iii. Admission, readmission and discharge rates in hospitals.
  iv. Stay duration in hospitals.
  v. Absence from school or work.
  vi. OPD attendance.

Q 14. Write a note on "concept of disease". (S. 97, 06, 09; W. 98, 00, 04, 05)

The term "disease" is defined by many ways:

- Disease is a physiological or psychological dysfunction.
- Disease is any deviation from normal state of complete physical, mental or social well-being.
- Disease is a condition of the body or some part or organ of the body in which its functions are disturbed.
- The WHO has not defined the disease because disease has many shades (spectrum of disease) ranging from subclinical cases to severe illness.

Q 15. Write a note on "natural history of disease". (S. 95, 02, 05, 06, 07; W. 96, 05, 07)

The term natural history of disease signifies the way in which a disease evolves over time from the earliest stage of pathogenesis phase to its termination as recovery, disability or death in the absence of treatment or prevention.

Disease results from a complex interaction between person, an agent (disease agent) and the environment.

Natural history of disease consists of two phases namely:

i. *Prepathogenesis phase*: It is the phase at which causative agent exists in the environment. In this phase, the man is exposed to the risk of disease.

   The causative factors of disease may be classified as agent, host and environment. These three factors are referred to as epidemiological triad.

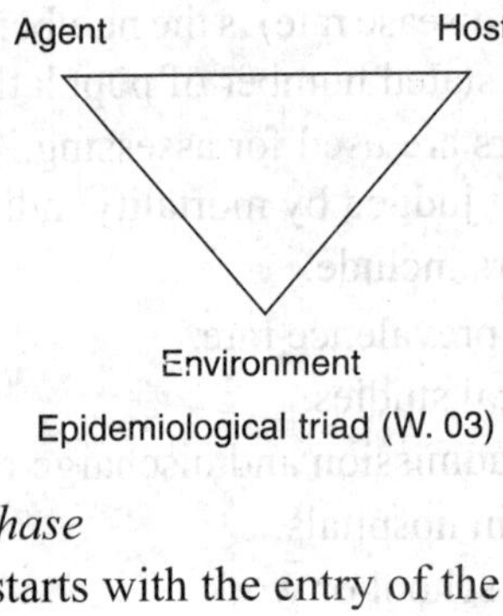

Epidemiological triad (W. 03)

ii. *Pathogenesis phase*
   - This phase starts with the entry of the agent into the human host.

- The time interval from the entry of agent in the host to the appearance of disease is termed as incubation period.
- During this period the agent multiplies in the host's tissues without producing symptoms of disease.
- The incubation period is followed by pathological changes in the form of early and late pathogenesis.

Q 16. Define the term "disease agent". Classify various disease agents. (S. 04, 06; W. 08)

Disease Agent

Disease agent is a substance living or nonliving or a force tangible or intangible the excessive presence or relative lack of which is the immediate cause of a particular disease.

The disease agents are classified as:

i. *Biological agents*: These are microorganisms including bacteria, viruses, fungi, protozoa.
ii. *Nutrient agents*: These include proteins, fats, carbohydrates, vitamins, minerals and water.
iii. *Physical agents*: These include heat, cold, humidity, radiation, electricity, pressure, sound.
iv. *Chemical agents*:
   - Endogenous, e.g. urea, bilirubin, uric acid, cholesterol.
   - Exogenous, e.g. pollens, fumes, gases, insecticides.
v. *Mechanical agents*: Vibration, chronic friction and other mechanical forces can lead to trauma.
vi. Absence or insufficiency or excess factors necessary for health may be the cause of disease, e.g. hormones, enzymes.
vii. *Social agents*: These include poverty, smoking alcohol, unhealthy lifestyles.

Q 17. Explain the "concepts of prevention of diseases". (S. 97, 99, 00, 01, 03, 04, 05, 07, 08; W. 98, 00)

The concept of prevention of diseases includes following three levels:

Primary Prevention

Primary prevention can be defined as "action taken prior to the onset of disease, which removes the possibility that disease will ever occur.

i. Primary prevention is exercised to promote general health and well-being and quality of life of the people.

ii. The concept of primary prevention is now being applied to the prevention of chronic disease like hypertension, cancer.
iii. Primary prevention is the safest and low cost way of prevention of disease.

Secondary Prevention

Secondary prevention can be defind as "actions which are taken to half the progress of a disease at its early stage and to prevent complications.

i. Secondary prevention arrest the disease process by early diagnosis and treatment.
ii. Secondary prevention is an important tool in the control of transmission of diseases.
iii. The health programs of government are usually at the level of secondary prevention.
iv. It is often more expensive and less effective than primary prevention.

Tertiary Prevention

Tertiary prevention can be defined as "all measures available to reduce or limit impairments and disabilities, minimise sufferings caused by existing departures from good health and to promote the patients adjustment to irremediable conditions".

Tertiary prevention includes disability prevention and rehabilitation of the patients.

Q 18. What is intervention? What are various modes of intervention?

Intervention

Any measure taken to intervene or interrupt the natural sequence of a disease is termed as intervention.

Intervention includes treatment, education, help or social support.

The modes of intervention are:

i. *Health promotion*: Health promotion is intended to strengthen the host by improving the general health and quality of life of individual and communities.
   The important interventions for health promotion are:
   – Health education
   – Environmental modifications

- Nutritional intervention
- Lifestyle and behavioural changes.

ii. *Specific protection*: It includes specific immunization, use of specific nutrients, protection against accidents, etc.

iii. *Early diagnosis and treatment*: Early detection and treatment are the main interventions of disease control.

iv. *Disability limitation*: The objective at this level is to control the disease process by appropriate treatment to limit the disability and further complications.
Disease → Impairment → Disability → Handicap

v. *Rehabilitation*: It is defined as "the combined and coordinated use of medical social, educational and vocational measures for training and retraining the individual to the highest possible level of functional ability". The important areas of rehabilitation are as follows:
- *Medical rehabilitation*: Restoration of function.
- *Vocational*: Restoration of the capacity to earn a livelihood.
- *Social*: Restoration of family and social relationship.
- *Psychological*: Restoration of personal dignity and confidence.

CHAPTER 2

Nutrition and Health

Q 1. Define the term "nutrition" and "food". Mention the functions of food. (S. 95, 96, 97, 02, 09; W. 96, 04, 05)

Nutrition

Nutrition is a process in which the food is utilized for nourishing the body.

WHO in 1971 defined nutrition as follows:

"It is the science of food and its relationship to health."

Food

A food may be defined as any substance which when taken into the body can be utilized to provide heat or energy to maintain and compensate wear and tear of the tissues and to regulate body processes.

Functions of Food

- It provides energy to the body in the form of heat for mechanical work.
- It is essential for the growth of the body and for the repair of damaged tissues.
- It is essential for maintenance and regulation of tissue functions and body temperature.
- It provides the power to the body to build resistance against infections and diseases.
- It is essential to satisfy hunger.

Q 2. Give the classification of food materials. (S. 97; W. 96, 04)

Classification of Food

- On the basis of function:
  i. Energy yielding foods, e.g. cereals sugars, roots, oils.

   ii. Body building foods, e.g. meat, egg, fish and pulses.
   iii. Protective foods, e.g. vegetables, fruits, milk.
- On the basis of origin:
   i. Animal origin, e.g. eggs, fish, meat.
   ii. Plant origin, e.g. vegetables, fruits.
   iii. Mineral origin, e.g. mineral salts.
- According to chemical composition:
   i. Carbohydrates
   ii. Proteins
   iii. Fats
   iv. Vitamins
   v. Minerals.
- On the basis of nutritive value:
   i. Cereals and millets (carbohydrates, proteins).
   ii. Pulses (proteins, minerals).
   iii. Vegetables (minerals, vitamins).
   iv. Fruits (minerals, vitamins).
   v. Animal foods (proteins, fats, vitamins).
   vi. Fats and oils (fats, vitamins A and D).
   vii. Sugar and jaggery (carbohydrates, iron).
   viii. Condiments and spices (act as carminatives and digestants).
   ix. Miscellaneous food articles.

Q 3. Define proteins. Give the sources and mention the functions of proteins. (S. 02, 05, 08; W. 99, 00, 01, 02, 03, 05, 08)

Proteins

"The proteins are complex organic nitrogenous compounds made up of amino acids and are necessary for overall growth and repair processes of body tissues."

Sources of Proteins

Fish, liver, meat, pulses, milk, egg, nuts, soya bean.

Functions of Proteins

- Proteins are required for body building.
- Repair and maintenance of body tissues.
- Maintenance of osmotic pressure.
- Synthesis of substances like plasma proteins haemoglobin.
- Production of heat and energy like carbohydrates.

Q 4. What do you mean by essential and nonessential amino acids? Give five examples of each.

Essential Amino Acids (S. 95, 07; W. 07, 08)

The amino acids which cannot be synthesized in the body but are badly required for normal functioning are called as essential amino acids, e.g. leucine, isoleucine, arginine, histidine, valine, phenylalanine.

Nonessential Amino Acids

The amino acids which are synthesized in the body but are not very essential for normal functioning are called nonessential amino acids, e.g. alanine, proline, tyrosine, glycine, cystine, serine.

Q 5. What are proteins? Give the classification of proteins giving suitable examples. (S. 96, 98, 02)

Proteins

The proteins are complex organic nitrogenous compounds made up of amino acids and are necessary for overall growth and repair processes of body tissues.

Classification of Proteins

Proteins

Simple proteins	Conjugated/complex proteins	Derived proteins
a. Albumins	a. Nucleoproteins	
b. Globulins	b. Phosphoproteins	
c. Glutelins	c. Glycoproteins	
d. Prolamins	d. Lipoproteins	
e. Protamines	e. Chromoproteins	
f. Histamines	f. Metalloproteins	

Q 6. What are amino acids? Classify them with examples. Mention the functions of amino acids. (S. 97, 98, 99, 00, 01)

Amino Acids

Amino acids are the building blocks of proteins.

Classification of Amino Acids

- Neutral amino acids, e.g. glycine, alanine, valine.
- Basic amino acids, e.g. lysine, arginine, histidine.

- Acidic amino acids, e.g. aspartic acid, glutamic acid.
- Imino acids, e.g. proline, hydroxyproline.

Functions of Amino Acids

- Amino acids are required for synthesis of various enzymes, hormones, plasma proteins and immunoglobulins.
- For growth and repair of body tissues.
- As a source of energy when body is having inadequate supply of carbohydrates or fats.

Q 7. What is kwashiorkor disease? Give its symptoms and mode of treatment. (S. 98, 00, 01, 08)

Kwashiorkor Disease

It is a protein deficiency disease occurring commonly in the children. It is characterized by qualitative and quantitative deficiency of proteins.

Causes/Contributory Factors of Kwashiorkor

- Large family size.
- Poor health of mother.
- Premature termination of breastfeeding.
- Poor environmental condition.
- Delayed supplementary feeding.
- Use of diluted cow's milk to the infants or children.

Symptoms/Effects of Kwashiorkor

- Retarded growth.
- Oedema.
- Changes or alteration in pigmentation of skin and hair.
- Changes in texture of skin.
- Enlargement of liver.
- Hypoalbuminaemia.
- GIT disturbances.
- Psychic changes.
- Hypoglycaemia.
- Stools containing much higher quantity of undigested food.

Other Symptoms

- Macrocytic anaemia.
- Normocytic anaemia.

- Decreased BMR.
- Fall in body temperature.
- Fall in plasma levels of triglycerides cholesterol.

Treatment for Kwashiorkor

- Supply of diet rich in protein.
- First choice milk and egg should be given both being rich in proteins.
- Soyabeans are best known vegetarian source of first class as well as second class proteins.
- Food from nonvegetarian source like liver, meat, sea food.
- In severe condition blood transfusions are required.
- The use of preventive measures is the best way for avoiding this disease.

Q 8. What is marasmus disease? Give its symptoms and treatments.

Marasmus Disease

It is the protein deficiency disease commonly found in infants below 1 year of age.

Causes

- It is mainly caused due to deficiency of proteins and carbohydrates with some other nutritional factors.
- Proteins and energy deficiency disease of such type is also known as marasmic kwashiorkor.
- It is commonly found in people in absence of maintaining proper diet.
- Early stop breastfeeding.

Symptoms

- Retarded growth.
- Complete loss of body fat.
- Weakness.
- Changes in texture of skin.
- GIT disturbances.
- Oedema.
- Alteration in pigmentation of skin and hair.

Treatments

- Providing diet rich in calories.
- Providing protein diet.

- Other nutritional factors is best course of prevention and cure of marasmus.

Q 9. What do you mean by complete and incomplete proteins? Give examples.

Complete Proteins

Proteins which contain all the essential amino acids in required quantities are called as complete proteins, e.g. milk proteins, egg proteins.

Incomplete Proteins

Proteins which do not contain all essential amino acids are called as incomplete proteins, e.g. gelatin, zein of maize.

Q 10. What is "malnutrition"? Explain protein-energy malnutrition (PEM). (S. 98, 99, 02, 06; W. 96, 97, 99, 02)

Malnutrition

Malnutrition is defined as the lack of necessary or proper food substances in the body or defective absorption and distribution of them.

Protein-energy Malnutrition (PEM)

- Protein-energy malnutrition (PEM) is supposed to be a major health problem in India.
- It is common among children during the first few years of life.

Causes of PEM

- Consumption of food inadequate in quantity and quality.
- Infections like diarrhoea, respiratory infections, intestinal worms.
- Decrease in absorption and utilization of proteins.

Clinically the protein-energy malnutrition is manifested in two forms:

i. Kwashiorkor disease ii. Marasmus disease.

Q 11. What are carbohydrates? Explain the role of carbohydrates in our food. (S. 05)

Carbohydrates

Carbohydrates are the compounds of carbon, hydrogen and oxygen and are chemically polyhydroxy aldehydes or ketones or compounds derived from them, e.g. glucose, fructose, galactose, sucrose, maltose, lactose, starch, cellulose.

Role of carbohydrates in our foods is:

i. *Cellulose*: It is a dietary fibre and important content and diet found in vegetables, fruits and grains.
   - It increases the bulk of stool and reduces the tendency for constipation.
   - These fibres also possess cholesterol lowering activity.
   - Excretion of minerals in stool is increased by high fibre diet.

ii. *Starch*: The largest proportion of carbohydrates in our diet occurs as starch. Plants store the greatest part of their food reserve as starch. The dietary sources of starch are cereals, potatoes, unripe fruits.

iii. *Glycogen*: It is the carbohydrate of animal origin which is deposited in liver and muscles. The glycogen reserve of human adult is about 500 grams.

Q 12. What are fats? Give the sources and functions of fats. OR Define and classify lipids. Give functions of lipids. (S. 01; W. 98)

Fats or Lipids

Fats or lipids are compounds of glycerol with fatty acids. Fats are solid up to 20°C and if they are liquid at that temperature are called as oils.

Sources of Fats/Lipids

Coconut oil, palm oil, cotton seed oil, ground nut oil, fish oil, sesame oil, soyabean oil.

Classification of Fats/Lipids

Fats/lipids

- Simple lipids
  - i. Oils and fats
  - ii. Waxes
- Compound lipids
  - i. Phospholipids
  - ii. Glycolipids
  - iii. Sulpholipids
  - iv. Lipoproteins
  - v. Lipopolysaccharides
- Derived lipids
  - i. Cholesterol
  - ii. Prostaglandins
- Others
  - i. Vit. E
  - ii. Vit. K
  - iii. Carotenoids

Functions of Fats/Lipids

- Fats are high energy foods (source of energy).
- Act as a vehicle for fat soluble vitamins like A, D, E, K.

- As an insulator of organs of cell.
- Building blocks for membranes.
- Support viscera like heart, kidneys and intestine.

Q 13. Define minerals. How are minerals classified? Give the basic functions of minerals. (S. 95, 00, 99, 03, 05, 06; W. 99, 00, 01)

Minerals

Minerals are various elements which are required for metabolic functions in the body, e.g. calcium, phosphorus, sodium, potassium, iron, iodine.

Classification/Types of Minerals

- *Macrominerals/macroelements/principle elements/macronutrients*: The minerals which are required in large quantities for human body with respect to daily requirement are called as macroelements, e.g. Ca, P, Na, K, Mg, Fe, Zn.
- *Microelements/microminerals/trace elements/micronutrients*: The minerals which are required in very less quantities (trace quantities) for the human body with respect to daily requirements are called as microminerals/trace elements, e.g. Co, Cu, I, Se, Mn.

Q 14. State the basic functions of minerals present in the body. (S. 00, 03; W. 99, 00, 01)

The minerals are needed for:

i. Maintenance of osmotic pressure of blood (Na^+, K^+, CT).
ii. Transport of oxygen (Fe).
iii. Growth and maintenance of tissues and bones (Ca^{++}).
iv. Working of nervous system (Ca^{++}).
v. Muscle contraction (Ca^{++}).
vi. Maintenance of electrolyte balance (Na^+, K^+).
vii. Acid-base balance.
viii. Blood coagulation (Ca^{++}).
ix. Cardiac activity (Ca^{++}).
x. Maturation of sperms (Zn).
xi. Thyroid hormone synthesis (I).

Q 15. Give the requirements, deficiency effects, sources and importance/functions of following minerals in human body.

	Minerals	*Sources*	*Requirements*	*Deficiency disorders*	*Functions/role/importance*
1.	Calcium	Milk, egg, leafy vegetables	Adults: 400–500 mg/day Infants and children 500–600 mg/day	Rickets, osteoporosis, hypocalcaemia osteomalacia tetany	i. For formation and maintenance of growth of bone ii. For formation of tooth iii. For blood clotting iv. For absorption of vitamin B_{12} v. For contraction of muscles vi. For activation of enzymes vii. For accessibility of nerve fibres
2.	Phosphorus	Food stuffs	Adult: 0.8 gm/day Infants/children: 0.2 to 0.3 gm/day	Hypophosphataemia, rickets, Osteomalacia	i. For formation of developments of bones and teeth ii. For formation of phospholipids, nucleic acids iii. It forms coenzymes like NADP, ADP, AMP, ATP iv. It is required in the absorption of glucose by phosphorylation
3.	Sodium	Fish, meat, milk, table salt	Adult: 10–15 gm/day	Hyponatremia, Addison's disease	i. For maintenance of osmotic pressure ii. For retaining water in the body iii. For neuromuscular junction activity

Contd...

Minerals	*Sources*	*Requirements*	*Deficiency disorders*	*Functions/role/importance*
				iv. For flexibility of nerves v . For acid-base balance vi. For maintenance of viscosity of blood vii. To maintain electrolyte balance
4. Iodine	Sea fish, cod liver oil, Sea weeds, milk, meat, cereals, vegetables	Adult: 50 gm/day	Goitre cretinism, hypothy-roidism	i. For biosynthesis of thyroid hormones ii. For growth and development of body
5. Iron	Liver, meat, poultry, fish, cereals, green leafy vegetables, nuts, jaggery, dry fruits	Adult: 2–6 gm/day	Iron deficiency, anaemia, Haemochromatosis	i. For treatment of anaemia ii. As a haematinic

Q 16. What are vitamins? How are they classified? (S. 95, 98, 99, 07, 08)

Vitamins

Vitamins are the organic compounds which are found in natural food stuffs and essential for normal growth and metabolic functions of the body.

Classification of Vitamins

- *Fat soluble vitamins*: Vitamins A, D, E, and K.
- *Water soluble vitamins*:
  i. Vitamin C (ascorbic acid)
  ii. Vitamin B complex:
    - Thiamine (B_1)
    - Riboflavin (B_2)
    - Niacin (B_3)
    - Pyridoxin (B_6)
    - Pantothenic acid
    - Biotin
    - Folic acid
    - Lipolic acid (PABA)
    - Cyanocobalamin (B_{12}).

Q 17. Give the sources, daily requirements, deficiency effects, role/functions of following vitamins. *See Table next page*

Q 18. What is balanced diet? Give the composition of balanced diet. What are the common deficiency/faults in Indian diet? (S. 97, 98, 99, 01, 02, 04; W. 00, 05, 06)

Balanced Diet

A balanced diet is defined as one which contains variety of foods in such quantities and proportions that the need for energy, amino acids, vitamins, minerals, fats, carbohydrates and other nutrients is adequately met for maintaining health, vitality and general well-being and also makes a provision for extranutrients to withstand short duration of leanness.

A balanced diet has become an accepted means to safeguard a population from nutritional deficiencies.

Vitamins	*Sources*	*Requirements per day*	*Deficiency effects*	*Role/functions*
1. Vitamin A	Fish, liver, butter ghee, whole milk, fish.	Adult: 750 µg Children: 250 to 600 µg	Night blindness, conjunctival xerosis, Bitot's spot, xerophthalmia	i. To maintain visual activities ii. Normal functioning of epithelial tissues and glands iii. Supports normal growth of skeleton iv. Anti-infective action
2. Vitamin D	Fish, liver oil animal fat	Adults: 25 µg Infant/children 5.00 µg	Rickets, osteomalacia	i. Promotes normal growth and development of bone ii. Promotes absorption of calcium and phosphorus iii. Allows maturation of collagen and collagenous tissue iv. It promotes overall normal growth of the body
3. Vitamin C	Fresh citrus fruits, green leafy vegetables, amla	Adult: 40 mg/day Infant/children: 40 mg/day	Scurvy	i. Helps to prevent skin lesions and infections like scurvy ii. Increases the resistance of the body against infection iii. Keeps the gums and teeth healthy iv. Necessary for normal tissue oxidation physiology v. Acts as a coenzyme

Contd...

Vitamins	*Sources*	*Requirements per day*	*Deficiency effects*	*Role/functions*
				vi. Required for absorption of iron vii. Helps in wound healing process
4. Vitamin B_1 (thiamine)	Yeast, pulses, oil seeds, nuts, cereals	0.5 mg/100 kcal/day	Beriberi, dry beriberi, wet beriberi, infantile beriberi, Cerebral beriberi	i. For the treatment of beriberi ii. Involved in synthesis of acetylcholine iii. Acts as a coenzyme
5. Vitamin B_2 (riboflavin)	Liver, meat, eggs, milk	0.6 mg/1000 kcal/day	Corneal ulcers, cataracts, photophobia	i. Acts as a coenzyme ii. Involved in metabolism of proteins, fats and carbohydrates iii. To treat a riboflavinosis
6. Niacin	Liver, ground nut, whole cereals, pulses meat, fish	6.6 mg/1000 kcal/day	Pellagra	i. In treatment of pellagra ii. As antihyperlipidemic agent iii. As a vasodilator iv. Essential for normal functioning of skin, intestine, etc.
7. Vitamin B_{12} (cyanoco-balamin)	Liver, kidney meat, fish, eggs, milk, cheese	Adult: 1 µg/day Children: 0.2 to 1 µg/day	Megaloblastic anaemia, pernicious anaemia	i. Required for normal development and maturation of RBC ii. As a coenzyme iii. Required for conversion of RNA into DNA

Composition of Balanced Diet

- Fats—20 to 30%.
- Carbohydrates—50–70%.
- Vitamins.
- Minerals.
- Proteins—meat, liver fish, milk, pulses.
- Foods rich in vitamins and minerals—milk, eggs, liver, fruits.
- Foods rich in carbohydrates and fats—cereals, sugar, roots, tubers.

In Indian diet common deficiencies are lower proteins, fats, carbohydrates, vitamins, amino acids and other substances which are essential for balanced diet.

In addition, a balanced diet should also contain sufficient amounts of water and roughage material.

The balanced diet (food) should satisfy the taste and desire of a person.

Q 19. Explain the terms.

a. Night Blindness

It is an inability to have vision in dimlight and during dark due to impairment in dark adaptation of eyes. It is caused due to deficiency of vitamin A.

In children, additional defects like recurrent infections and diarrhoea may be observed.

b. Pellagra

It is caused due to deficiency of niacin (vitamin B_3).

Symptoms

i. Dermatitis
ii. A sore
iii. Dark-coloured tongue
iv. An inability to digest and assimilate food
v. Skin rash, itching.

c. Scurvy (W. 00, 01)

It is deficiency disorder caused due to vitamin C.

Symptoms

i. Defective formation of collagen fibres of connective tissues.
ii. Formation of bone is also abnormal.

iii. Bleeding occurs.
iv. Pin-point haemorrhages in the skin.
v. Bleeding from gums and teeth.
vi. Slow wound healing
vii. Slow healing of fractured bones.

d. Egg White Injury

It is a deficiency disorder caused due to vitamin 'biotin'. Biotin has a strong affinity with avidin (egg white protein). Excess consumption of raw eggs results in deficiency of biotin called as egg white injury.

This biotin-avidin complex is not absorbed during digestion and hence produces deficiency of biotin.

Symptoms

i. Nausea
ii. Anorexia
iii. Dermatitis
iv. Pains in muscles
v. Fatigue.

e. Beriberi (S. 97; W. 97, 07, 08)

It is a deficiency disorder of vitamin B_1 (thiamine). There are four types of beriberi.

i. *Dry beriberi*: It is a nutritional deficiency. The main reason behind this is consumption of polished rice and refined cereals.
Symptoms
   - Degeneration and demyelination.
   - Edema of face and legs.
   - Pericardial pains.
   - Palpitation.
   - Numbness in legs.
   - Tenderness in the calf muscles.

ii. *Wet beriberi*: It is mainly characterized by edema. Reason behind edema is cardiac failure.
Symptoms
   - Rapid and notable edema develops involving face, legs, trunk and serous cavities.
   - Breathlessness.
   - Palpitation.
   - Rise in systolic BP.

– In severe condition patient may die due to acute circulatory failure.

iii. *Infantile beriberi*: It occurs in breastfed infants, usually between 2 to 5 months of age. Reason behind is mother consuming thiamine-deficient diet and secreting milk with low thiamine content. It is very acute condition and can be fatal (toxic).

Symptoms

– Restlessness in infants.
– Infant cries a lot and passes very less urine.
– Edema develops.
– Dysphonia.
– Tachycardia.
– Infant may die within 24 to 48 hours.
– Convulsion and coma.

iv. *Cerebral beriberi*: This disease is resultant of acute biochemical lesions in the brain due to thiamine-deficient diet. It is further leading to abnormal metabolism in the brain.

Reasons behind cerebral beriberi

– Alcoholism.
– Carcinoma in stomach.
– Pregnancy toxaemia.
– Prolonged vomiting.
– Diarrhoea.

Symptoms

– Vomiting.
– Psychiatric disorders like disorientation, faulty memory.
– Loss of pupillary reflex.
– Loss of extraocular movements.
– Polyneuritis.

Q 20. Discuss in brief various nutrition-related programmes developed by government of India. (W. 02)

The government of India has developed various nutrition-related programmes to counter the problem of malnutrition in India. These programmes are as follows:

i. *Vitamin A prophylaxis programme*: It helps for the control of blindness and involves administration of a single massive dose of oily preparation of vitamin A containing 200,000 IU.

ii. *Prophylaxis against nutritional oedema*: It involves distribution of iron and folic acid tablets.

iii. *Control of iodine deficiency disorders*: It involves replacement of edible salt by iodized salt.

iv. *Special nutrition programmes*: It was started for the benefit of children below 6 years of age, pregnant and nursing mothers in urban slums, tribal areas and backward rural areas.

v. *Balwadi nutrition programme*: It is mainly for children in the age group of 3 to 6 years in rural areas.

vi. *Mid-day meal programme*: Its objective is to attract more children to schools and retain them. It involves providing them balanced diet.

Q 21. What is ORS/ORT? Give its composition and mention its uses. (S. 03)

ORS/ORT means 'oral rehydration salt' or 'oral rehydration therapy'.

- These are orally administered electrolyte solutions used to supply water and electrolytes needed to the patients.
- Composition of ORS/ORT

i. Sodium chloride	3.5 gm
ii. Potassium chloride	1.5 gm
iii. Sodium bicarbonate	2.5 gm
iv. Glucose	20 gm

- This mixture is added in 1 litre of water and then taken by oral route.
- Uses of ORS/ORT: It is the first aid remedy in condition of dysentery, diarrhoea, prolonged fever, vomiting, etc.

CHAPTER 3

Demography and Family Planning

Q 1. Define "demography". Give the objectives of study of population. (S. 04, 06; W. 05, 08)

Demography

Demography is the scientific study of the human population.

Objectives of Demography

- To study the change in population size.
- To study the composition of population.
- To study the distribution of population in space.

Q 2. Define demographic cycle. Explain stages of demographic cycle. (S. 96, 97, 00, 03, 05; W. 97, 99, 02, 05)

Demographic Cycle

"The cycle which suggests the population growth of nation is known as demographic cycle."

Five stages of demographic cycle are as follows:

i. *First stage* (*high stationary stage*)
   - It is the first sage through which nation begins.
   - At this stage birth rate is very high as well as death rate is also very high. Hence there is no increase in population size.
   - India was in this stage up to 1920.

ii. *Second stage* (*early expanding stage*)
   - In this stage death rate was decreased while birth rate was not affected so the population started increasing.
   - In some countries birth rate was increased due to improved health care facilities.
   - Many African and Asian countries are passing through this stage.

  - As the population has started increasing this stage is also called 'early expanding stage'.

iii. *Third stage* (*late expanding stage*)
  - In this stage death rate continues to fall and birth rate also started to decrease.
  - Therefore, population continues to increase.
  - Many developing countries like China, Singapore are in this stage.

iv. *Fourth stage* (*low stationary stage*)
  - In this stage population is stabilized.
  - The low death rate and low birth rate results in constant population (stable).
  - It is also called as zero population growth.

v. *Fifth stage* (*declining*)
  - In this stage population decreases because birth rate is lower than death rate.

Q 3. What is fertility? Explain factors affecting fertility. (S. 96, 99, 00, 01, 06, 07; W. 96, 99)

Fertility

Fertility means the actual bearing of children.

A woman's reproductive period is from 15 to 45 years.

Factors affecting/influencing Fertility

Factors on which fertility depends are:

- *Age of marriage*: Earlier the marriages, higher is the level of fertility. Females who are marrying later have fewer number of children.
- *Duration of married life*: All the efforts towards fertility control should be within 10–15 years of married life of the couple because the majority of births take place during this period.
- *Spacing of children*: Spacing methods are properly advised to females of 25–30 years to have fertility control.
- *Education*: Well educated females give births to less number of children than uneducated females.
- *Economic status*: When economic condition of the family is good, more attention is given to control fertility.
- *Religions and caste*: Muslims and lower caste Hindus have comparatively higher fertility.

- *Nutrition*: All poorly fed communities have higher fertility rates.
- *Family planning*: It is the most important key factor in decreasing fertility in most of the developed countries.
- *Other factors*: Fertility is affected by the number of physical, social, biological and cultural factors such as value of children in society, breastfeeding, customs and beliefs, better health conditions and housing.

Q 4. Write a note on family welfare programme. (S. 98, 99, 00, 01, 02, 09; W. 98, 00, 02)

- The term 'family welfare' is now used in place of the 'family planning'.
- Family welfare signifies "the improvement of the quality of health and welfare of the entire family".
- Family welfare includes:
  i. Spacing and limitation of birth.
  ii. Advice on sterility.
  iii. Education of parenthood.
  iv. Sex education.
  v. Genetic counselling.
  vi. Carrying out pregnancy test.
  vii. Services to unmarried mothers.
  viii. Premarital examination and counselling.
  ix. Maternity and child health services.
  x. Immunisation service.
- Before 1970 the family welfare programme advocated 2 to 3 children in a family.
- In 1980, they advocated only 2 child norms.
- In 1990, they say that whether daughter or son is enough.
- The department of family welfare has increased the interaction with state government for improving the quality of family welfare programme.

Objectives of Family Welfare Programme

- Reduction in the number of children by only one in family shows remarkable effect on growth rate of whole country.
- It helps to promote on a voluntary basis for controlling number of children.

- To raise decision-making capabilities in taking care of their reproductive health, number of children.
- It helps to educate and to make awareness in the mothers to control the number of children in the family.

Q 5. Write a note on population explosion/population problem in India. (S. 03, 09; W. 06)

Population Problem/Population Explosion in India

India faces a serious population problem which is ever increasing. This is due to an increase in the birth rate and decrease in the death rate.

The death rate has decreased because of new inventions and better developments in the science and medicine. Hence most of the diseases can be cured, as a result death rate decreases. Whereas birth rate has not decreased to keep a balance in the population. The increase in birth rate is due to child marriage mainly in rural areas. This may be due to lack of knowledge about the advantages of family planning.

Due to the population increase, the economy of the country does not show progress as all effects are concentrated on fighting against the poverty, due to this population increases. As a result, there is no progress in any other important field.

Therefore, it is necessary to control population increase by accepting family planning at a national level for the progress of our country.

The government of India has made family planning as a national policy.

Q 6. Define the term "family planning". Give the objectives of family planning. (S. 96, 97, 99, 05, 06, 08; W. 97, 99, 04, 07)

Family Planning

Family planning means to decide "the number and timings of children in the family" in its simplest sense.

WHO defined family planning as "a way of living and thinking that is adopted voluntarily, upon the basis of knowledge, attitude and responsible decisions by individuals and couples in order to promote the health and welfare of the family group and thus contribute effectively to social development of a country".

Objectives/Importance/Advantages/Merits of Family Planning

- To avoid unwanted births.
- To bring about wanted births.

- To regulate the intervals between pregnancies.
- To control the time at which birth occurs in relation to ages of the parents.
- To determine the number of children in the family.
- To preserve the health of the mother, the welfare of the child and give happiness at home.
- To control the population problem.

Q 7. Define contraceptives and contraception. Classify methods of contraception/family planning. (S. 97, 99, 02, 04, 05, 06, 07, 08; W. 00, 01, 02, 08)

Contraceptives (S. 06, 09; W. 07)

Contraceptives are the devices which restrict the fertility of ovum and do not allow the zygote formation. Or the devices which prevent the entry of sperm into uterus of the female to prevent pregnancy.

Contraception

"The prevention of pregnancy or to plan the pregnancy by using contraceptive devices is called as contraception."

Methods of Family Planning/Contraception

a. *Temporary Methods (Spacing Methods)*

i. Barrier methods
  - *Physical methods*:
    - Condom for male
    - Diaphragms, vaginal sponge for female.
  - *Chemical methods*: Foam tablets, creams, suppositories, jellies and pastes.

ii. Intrauterine devices (IUDs)
  - Medicated IUDs
  - Nonmedicated IUDs.

iii. Hormonal methods
  - Oral pills
  - Slow released preparations, e.g. vaginal rings, implants.

iv. Postconception methods
  - Menstrual regulation
  - Menstrual induction
  - Abortion.

v. Natural methods (miscellaneous methods)
   - Abstinence
   - Coitus interruption
   - Safe period (rhythm method)
   - Cervical mucus method.

b. *Permanent Methods/Terminal Methods/Sterilization Methods*

i. Male sterilization (vasectomy)
ii. Female sterilization (tubectomy)
iii. Laparoscopy.

Q 8. Explain physical method of contraception. OR Give the merits and demerits of (i) condom, (ii) diaphragm and capsule. (S. 96, 98, 00, 01; W. 97, 01, 02, 05, 07, 08)

Condom (Nirodh)

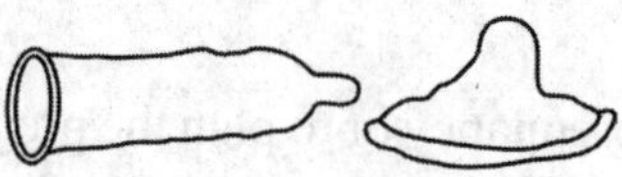

- It is a commonly used contraceptive device by male all over the world.
- It prevents pregnancy by preventing the deposition of semen in vagina.
- The condom is fitted on the erect penis before intercourse.

Advantages

- Easy to use and easily available.
- They are cheap and no medical supervision required.
- They are safe, used to protect sexually transmitted diseases.
- No side effect.
- Light, compact, disposable.

Disadvantages

- May slip off or tear during coitus.
- May interfere the sexual enjoyment of sexual intercourse.
- It is not 100% efficient.
- It is used only once a time.
- Possible to burst the condom.
- Many men do not use them regularly and carefully.

Diaphragms and Caps

There are the vaginal barriers made up of synthetic rubber or plastic. These devices close off the entrance of womb. These are inserted into the vagina and are fixed on the cervix before intercourse and must remain in place for not less than 6 hours after sexual intercourse.

Advantages

- These are reliable.
- No risks and side effects.
- Do not interfere with sexual pleasure.
- They are easy to handle and cheap.

Disadvantages

- Initially training by physician is needed to learn insertion of diaphragm.
- It is difficult to determine the size which fits the woman well.
- It requires careful attention to wash it, dry it, store it and protect it.
- In some cases diaphragm may be pushed away by the penis.
- Some women have allergy to diaphragm and cap.

Q 9. Write a note on chemical method of contraception.

Chemical Contraception

The purpose of using chemical contraceptives is to stop the sperms' progress completely or kill them before entering into the uterus of the female.

These contraceptives contain spermicide which kill the sperms.

i. *Foam tablets*: These are kept into vagina for 5 minutes before intercoitus. At body temperature they melt and produce a foam which acts as a barrier for the entry of sperms into uterus.

ii. *Pastes and jellies*: These are pushed into vagina with the help of applicator called as jelly applicator.

   Sufficient time is to be given to spread the chemical on the mouth of the uterus.

iii. *Soluble tablets*: These are kept into vagina for 5 minutes before intercoitus. At body temperature, they melt and spread the chemical on the mouth of uterus which kills the sperms.

Advantages of Chemical Contraceptives

- These are easy to obtain and simple to use.
- They are reliable and give good sexual satisfaction.
- Some chemicals also have lubricating action.

Disadvantages of Chemical Contraceptives

- High failure rates.
- Must be used immediately before intercourse.
- Some products can cause itching, burning and uneasiness.
- Some people do not like perfumes used in pastes and jellies.
- Foam tablets should be checked before use with the help of water.
- These devices should be used only once.
- Simple chemical barriers are not reliable hence they must be used with physical barriers such as condoms, caps.

Q 10. Write a note on IUCDs. (S. 96, 02, 07, 08; W. 99, 01)

Intrauterine Devices (IUDs) Intrauterine Contraceptive Devices (IUCDs)

These are devices placed in the uterus of women for preventing the pregnancy. These are highly reliable. They prevent implantation of fertilized ovum in the uterus.

The various IUDs include (types):

i. First generation IUDs, e.g. Lippes loop.
ii. Second generation IUDs, e.g. Copper-T, Nova-T.
iii. Third generation IUDs, e.g. Progestasert.

i. *First generation IUDs*: They are inert, nonmedicated devices made-up of polyethylene or other polymers. They appear in various shapes and sizes like loops, spirals, coils, springs, etc.

Lippes loop is commonly used device.

Lippes-loop: It is a double S-shaped device having nylon thread attached to it. The S-shaped loop is lined by polyethylene plastic material.

It does not require hospitalization for insertion.

A nylon thread is connected to other end which projects into the vagina. The falling of threads into vagina assures that loop is in place properly.

Advantages of Lippes loop

- Simple and easy insertion.
- Does not interfere with sexual pleasure.

- Cheap and safe.
- Reversible method.
- Can be used for a long time.

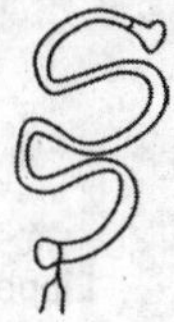

Lippes loop

Disadvantages of Lippes loop

- Needs a trained person for insertion.
- Should be replaced periodically (2 years).
- Needs adequate follow-up.
- Rarely it can produce cancer of uterus.

ii. *Second generation IUDs*: The second generation IUDs are copper-containing devices. Older devices are copper-T, copper-7, copper-T 200. Newer devices are Nova-T, multiload devices. Copper has antifertility effect. These devices release copper into uterus. Copper enhances cellular response in endometrium and alters the composition of cervical mucosa. The copper ions may affect sperm motility and survival.

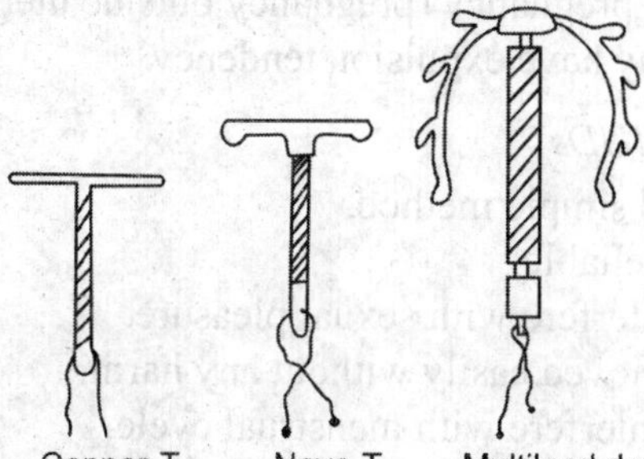

Copper-T Nova-T Multiload device

Advantages of second generation IUDs

- Low expulsion rate.
- Lower incidence of side effects like pain and bleeding.
- Easy to fit.
- Increased contraceptive effects.
- Can be kept for a long time.

iii. *Third generation IUDs (hormone releasing IUDs)*: These devices act by releasing a hormone in the uterus. The currently used device is 'Progestasert'. It is a T-shaped device filled progesterone, a natural hormone. It has a direct local effect on uterine lining, cervical mucus and sperms.

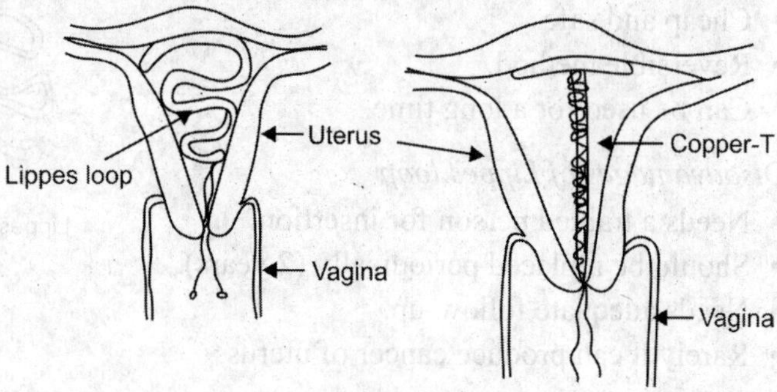

Position of IUDs

– Complications and side effects of IUDs:
  - Vaginal bleeding.
  - Pain in pelvis.
  - Pelvic infection.
  - Uterine perforation by IUD.
  - Pregnancy may occur in 3–5 per 100 IUD users per year.
  - Ectopic pregnancy (pregnancy outside uterus).
  - IUD may have expulsion tendency.

Advantages of IUDs

- It is safe and simple method.
- It is highly reliable.
- It will not interfere with sexual pleasure.
- It can be removed easily without any harm.
- It does not interfere with menstrual cycle.
- Insertion does not require hospitalization and requires only a few minutes.
- It is noncorrosive and nonirritant.
- It can be X-rayed to find its position.
- Once it is fitted, it is effective for years.
- Contraceptive effect is reversible.
- Free from systemic side effects.
- Highest acceptability.
- It does not affect the penis at the time of intercourse.

Disadvantages of IUDs

- It can produce heavy menstruation and pain in pelvis.
- It causes pains during insertion and after insertion.
- It may cause cramps and increased menstrual flow.

- Some women are unable to keep the IUD in place and can expel it out.
- It may cause side effects such as headache, bleeding from vagina, etc.
- It may cause cancer.
- It is not 100% efficient.

Q 11. Write a note on hormone contraceptives/oral contraceptives. (S. 96, 00, 01, 04, 08; W. 96, 97, 98, 03, 06)

Hormonal Contraceptives/Oral Contraceptives (Pills)

- Hormonal contraceptives are chemical agents in the form of tablets.
- These tablets make the women unable to ovulate.
- These contraceptives are almost 100% effective if taken properly. Oral and injectable preparations are available.
- These contraceptives contain a combination of both oestrogen and progesterone or progesterone only.
- In some packets, 28 pills are supplied.
- A woman has to take one pill per day starting from the 5th day of menstruation cycle.
- These pills prevent formation of matured ovum, i.e. prevent ovulation. Action may be due to formation of very thin endometrium, which is unable to grow fertilized ovum.
- Classification of hormonal contraceptives:
  - i. *Oral pills*
    - Combined pills
    - Progesterone only pill (POP)—minipills
    - Postcoital pill
    - Once a month pill
    - Male pill (under study).
  - ii. *Depot formulations* (slow released)
    - Injectable
    - Subcutaneous implants
    - Vaginal rings.

These hormonal contraceptives contain one or more different sex hormones.

i. *Oral Pills*

- *Combined pills*: Most of the combined pills contain oestrogen and progesterone.

The department of family welfare has made available two types of pills:
- Mala-N
- Mala-D

– *Progesterone only pills* (POP): POPs contain only progesterone which is given in small doses throughout cycle.

ii. *Depot formulations*
- Injectable formulations, e.g. depot methoxy progesterone acetate (DMPA).
- Subcutaneous implants, e.g. silastic capsules are implanted in the skin of the forearm.

Advantages of hormonal/oral contraceptives
- It is simple and easy method.
- Effectiveness up to 100%.
- It is most reliable method.
- Once, it is prescribed, it is not necessary to consult the doctor.
- It does not interfere with sexual pleasure.

Disadvantages of oral contraceptives
- These pills may cause side effects such as headache, pains in pelvis, unhealthy feeling and increse in body weight.
- Bleeding between the menstruation periods occurs.
- Nausea, breast tenderness.
- Increase in sugar and fat in blood.
- It may increase blood pressure.
- Pills may cause cancer.
- Reduced breast milk production.
- A woman has to take one pill per day starting from 5th day of menstruation.
- Pills should not be stopped between the days.
- Return to fertility may be developed.

Q 12. Explain natural methods of family planning. (S. 01, 03; W. 98, 99)

a. Abstinence

It is completely effective method but it is practically not possible to avoid the coitus by a couple.

b. Coitus Interruption (Withdrawal of Penis)

The principle of this method is the male withdraws his penis before ejaculation and prevents deposition of semen into vagina.

Disadvantages

- It gives sexual unsatisfaction to both partners.
- It is not reliable method because small amount of lubricating fluid which enters into vagina may contain sperms.
- It keeps strain on man's self-control.

c. Safe Period or Rhythm Method (S. 98, 01, 03, 04, 09; W. 98, 99)

This is also known as 'calender method'. One week before menstruation and one week after menstruation is considered as a safe period. During these days ovulation does not occur and conception can be avoided.

Advantages

- It is a natural means of birth control.
- It does not require an artificial means.

Disadvantages

- It is not reliable.
- It is difficult to find out safe period for a particular woman whose menstruation period changes.
- It requires arithmetic calculations.
- Many times there is no cooperation between the sexes.
- To be used by only educated and responsible couples.
- High failure rates.
- Ectopic pregnancies.
- Embryonic abnormalities.

Q 13. Explain permanent/terminal methods of sterilization. (S. 03, 06; W. 96, 01, 03, 08)

Permanent or Terminal Methods of Sterilization (Terminal Sterilization)

Sterilization Methods of Family Planning

This method involves surgical operations for both sexes. The methods are suitable for male of 25–40 years or female of 20 to 45 years of age.

i. *Male sterilization* (*vasectomy*): The surgical operation in case of male is known as vasectomy.

In this small operation, a small cut is taken on vas deferens or deferent ducts. The ducts are cut and their open ends are tied or ligated. Sometimes the open ends are turned away from one another.

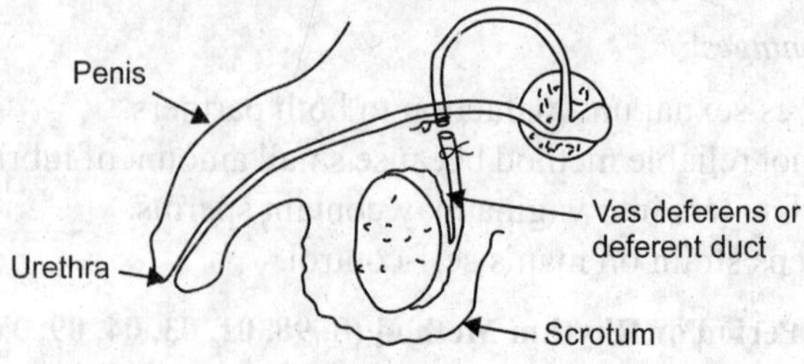

Vasectomy (male sterilization)

As the deferent ducts are cut and tied, the sperms from the testis are not carried towards urethra. Hence semen fluid ejaculated will not contain any sperm. Thus it prevents conception.

After the operation man should use other contraceptive methods during coitus such as condom at least for two months.

Disadvantages

- Possibility of infection.
- Granuloma of testis is possible.

ii. *Female sterilization* (*tubectomy*): The surgical operation in case of female is known as tubectomy.

In this operation, both the fallopian tubes are cut and tied. So that ovum cannot reach the uterus and thus no fertilization. The operation is major one and needs hospitalization. With the help of an instrument called laparoscope, the operation is performed within 2 to 3 minutes.

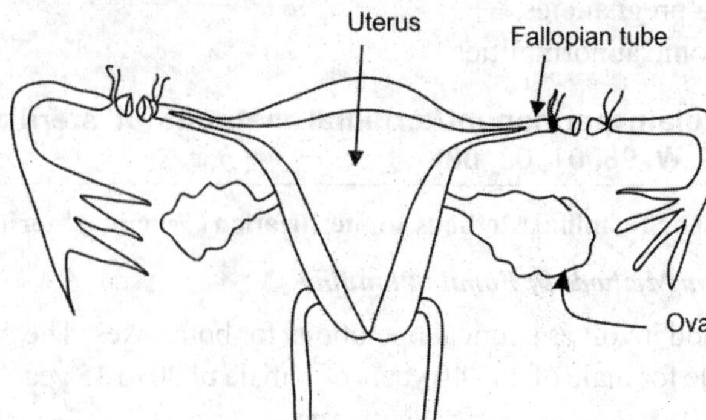

Tubectomy (female sterilization)

Q 14. Explain the role of pharmacist in promoting family planning. (S. 95, 99, 00, 01, 02; W. 98, 00, 02, 06, 07)

Role of Pharmacist in promoting Family Planning

- Pharmacist can maintain a reliable supply of contraceptives with a choice of methods and brands.
- Pharmacist can learn about family planning and advise customers accurately and actively.
- Pharmacist can set up self-service displays of condoms, spermicidal and oral contraceptives.
- Pharmacist can distribute brochures about family planning and display family planning posters.
- Pharmacist can work with other medical professionals to promote family planning.
- Pharmacist can advise a woman to consult a doctor before giving oral contraceptives, especially in known diabetic or hypertensive persons.
- Pharmacist can support the development of contraceptive social marketing programmes.
- Pharmacist can promote the image of the pharmacist as a provider of family planning supplies and information.
- Pharmacist can work with pharmacist's organizations to encourage their members to promote family planning.

CHAPTER 4

First Aid

Q 1. What is first aid? What are the basic objects/major principles of first aid? (S. 96, 97, 98, 00, 04, 05, 06, 07, 08; W. 96, 98, 02, 03, 06, 07)

First Aid

The first aid is the immediate treatment given to the patient or victim of an accident or sudden illness, till the patient is hospitalized.

Objects/Principles of First Aid

- To preserve life of the patient.
- To prevent further injury to the patient.
- To put injured person under medical cover at the earliest.
- Maintenance of respiration.
- To control haemorrhage.
- Prevention of shock.
- To avoid serious damage to the patient.

Q 2. Define resuscitation. What is cardiopulmonary resuscitation (CPR)? Explain ABC formula for CPR. Explain artificial respiration. (S. 98. 99, 02, 07, 08, 09; W. 99, 00, 01, 04, 08)

Resuscitation

It is defined as restoration of one's life, who is apparently dead (collapsed or ill shocked).

- First aid for unconscious patient, i.e. CPR. It means cardiopulmonary resuscitation.
- ABC formula for CPR: It is a type of first aid treatment given to unconscious patients. It mainly includes:
  i. Mouth to mouth artificial respiration.

ii. Mouth to nose respiration.
iii. Cardiac or chest massage.

- Care to be taken before starting ABC formula for CPR.
  i. Do not give water or tea, coffee to the victim as oral drink.
  ii. Never keep pillow under the head of the unconscious patients.
  iii. Putting a pillow below the legs helps to increase blood supply to chest and head.
  iv. Never move the patient or its body parts if there is a fracture or dislocation of bones.
  v. After observing all the points, CPR should be started immediately.

  The CPR can be done by ABC formula:

  'A' stands for airway.

  'B' stands for breathing.

  'C' stands for cardiac massage/chest massage/circulation.

'A' Stands for Airway

- First of all airway of patient should be opened and cleaned.
- By wrapping handkerchief, mouth of the patient is cleaned.
- Change the position of his face so that the airway is not blocked due to tongue which can fall backward.
- Keep the patient in his position with the chin facing upwards.
- Crowding surrounding the victim must be avoided.
- Increase the ventilation by operating doors and windows if the patient is in room. This allows circulation of clean and fresh air in the room, in the benefit of patient.

'B' Stands for Breathing

- A person may live without food for 70 days or can survive without water for 7 days but cannot survive more than 3 minutes without oxygen.
- If breathing is stopped then after cleaning, immediately start giving mouth to mouth breathing, also known as artificial breathing.
- This breathing can be done by closing tightly the nose of the patient by first two fingers and forcing lungful of air by mouth to mouth.
- The expansion of chest should be observed confirming entry of air into the lung. For adult, such 15 artificial breathings should be given in one minute.

- Mouth to nose respiration: If due to fracture of jaw, the patient cannot open the jaw, the mouth to nose respiration is used. In such case mouth of patient should be kept closed.

***'C' Stands for Chest Massage* (*Cardiac Massage*)**

- If it is found that the pulse of patient is missing, it is indication of failure of function of heart.
- In such situation cardiac massage is started.
- Cardiac massage is performed by pressing the chest by both the hands and by the hills of hand only.
- Pressure should be exerted in two fingers above the lower end of the sternum.
- While applying the pressure arm should be exactly perpendicular to area of compression.
- The pressure applied should be 10 kg/cm^2 or 20 pounds/inch^2 by which chest get pressed by 1.5 to 5 cm. By this way pressure is applied 60 to 80 times/min.
- If one is alone is performing CPR by above method, after every 50 compression, two is mouth to mouth or mouth to nose respiration should be given. But if two person are following CPR by above method, after every 5 compressions one artificial respiration should be given.

Q 3. Explain Silvester method/chest pressure arm lift method of artificial respiration. (W. 96, 02, 03)

- Place the victim on his back. Insert the support under his shoulder to raise them and allow his head to drop backward.
- Kneel at victim's head, keep the victims hand on the chest by crossing them over the lower chest part. The pressure should cause the air to flow out from victims nose and mouth.
- Immediately pull the arms outward and upward over his head and backward as far as possible. This should cause the inspiration.
- Repeat the whole cycle about 12 times a minute.
- If second rescuer is available, ask him to hold victims head so that the jaw will be in open condition.
- Any content of the mouth should be removed to keep mouth as clean as possible at all times.

Q 4. Describe Holger-Nielsen method or back pressure arm lifted method of artificial respiration. (S. 03, 04)

- Place the victim's face down with one hand on the other and turn his head slightly to one side and ensure that the jaw is opened.
- Kneel at the victim's head looking towards his feet. Place your hands to his back so that the palms lie just below the line or armpits.
- Apply a steady even pressure, downwards upon your hands.
- Immediately pull the arms upward and downward until you feel enough resistance and tension at his shoulder.
- Lower the arm and repeat the whole cycle of events about 12 times a minute.
- If second rescuer is available, then ask him to hold victim's head so that the jaw is in open condition.
- Remove contents of mouth if any and keep the mouth as clean as possible.

Q 5. Describe the first aid treatment in burns and scalds. (S. 95, 97, 01, 02, 04, 07, 08, 09; W. 97, 00, 01, 04, 08)

- Burns are the injuries caused by heat, fire, flames, electricity.
- Scalds are caused by moist heat due to boiling water, steam, oil and coal tar.
- Burns are classified as superficial burns, or deep burns depending upon the depth of tissue damage.
- Burns results into partial or complete skin loss.
- *First aid in burns*: The aim of first aid treatment of burns are:
    i. *Prevent further damage*
        - Remove the cause of burn from the casualty.
        - Burns should be treated immediately by showering in cold water.
        - Cooling prevents severity of burns and also relieves pains.
        - Cooling should be continued until no further relief from pain is produced.

    ii. *Prevent infection*
        - To prevent infection, the burnt area is quickly covered with a sterile dressing.
        - Clean, unused and well washed handkerchief, sheets or pillow covers are good to replace dressings.
        - Do not use cotton wool for the dressing of burns.

- Do not burst the blisters and do not apply any lotion or grease over the area.

iii. *Minimise the effects of loss of fluid from the burnt tissue*
- In burn cases the seriously damaging effects results due to fluid loss in greater volume.
- If the burnt casualty is conscious, give ample of water as oral drinks, weak tea or milk frequently until its hospitalization.

iv. *Reassure the burnt person*
- The assurance should be for making the victim calm and to make causalty as comfortable as possible.
- Relieve the anxiety of the patient by assuring him that he is in good hands.

v. *Transport of casualty to hospital*
- Send the patient to the hospital without delay.
- The patient should be given of fluids orally even during his journey to hospital.

Q 6. Describe emergency treatment in case of snakebite. (S. 96, 98, 99, 03, 06; W. 96, 98, 02, 05, 06, 07, 08)

- Out of 3500 species of snakes only 250 are poisonous.
- The viper, cobra, pit viper are found in all parts of world including India.
- All the sea snakes are poisonous.
- In cobra snake bite symptoms seen are: The patient feel sleepy, weakness of legs and gradually develops into paralysis of legs, excessive salivation, paralysis of tongue and pharynx produce difficulty in swallowing and speech. Patient may enter in coma and finally respiration and heart stops working.
- In viper snake poisoning symptoms seen are: Swelling and pains in bite area, abdominal pains, vomiting, complete loss of consciousness, increased body temperature. Bleeding may occurs from gums, rectum and site of bite. Death occurs due to shock and haemorrhage.
- *First aid treatment of snakebite*

  i. Assure the patient for his or her life being saved.

  ii. Apply very firm pressure over area of snake bite to avoid or delay poison circulation and absorption.

  iii. Tourniquet is used to prevent the blood flow towards the heart. Loosen the tourniquets for few seconds every 15 minutes.

iv. Immobilize the injured part, because mobility increases circulation of poison and so absorption of poison.
v. Make a cross incisions 1 cm long and 0.5 cm deep over each bite mark and allowed to bleed. Suck out the poison from wound and spit it out.
vi. Clean the wound with sterile saline or clean water and cover it with sterile dressing.
vii. If breathing is insufficient, then mouth to mouth artificial breathing should be practised.
viii. If cardiac failure is seen, heart massage also should be tried immediately.
ix. Intravenous or intramuscular administration of polyvalent antivenom should be given under medical supervision.
x. Patient should be shifted to a hospital as early as possible.

Q 7. Define shock. Mention different types of shock. Describe the first aid treatment for shock. (S. 95, 97, 01, 03, 05, 08; W. 99, 00, 01, 03)

Shock

Shock is rapidly developing syndrome caused by inadequate capillary perfusion of vital tissues.

- It is seen in conditions like heart attacks and strokes.
- Reasons for shock are: Multiple fractures, internal tissue damage, haemorrhage, serious head injury, chest injury, abdominal injury, poisoning, disturbances in CVS function, etc.

Types of Shock

- *Cardiac shock*: Due to heart disease.
- *Hypovolemic shock*: Due to dehydration, loss of blood or plasma.
- *Neurogenic shock*: Due to spinal cord injury.
- *Bacteremia shock*: Due to severe infections.
- *Haemo-obstructive shock*: Due to blockade of a main blood vessels.
- *Anaphylactic shock*: Due to injection of penicillin (allergic).

Emergency Treatment for Shock

- Keep the victim quite and lying down and elevate the legs to increases venous return to the heart.
- If bleeding is observed it should be arrested.
- Loosen clothings.

- If internal organs are not damaged then give some hot liquid orally as a tea or coffee.
- Keep the patient warm by providing blanket or rug.
- Do not rub any body part for warming purpose.
- Fear can take the patient in worst condition, so encourage the patient.
- Continuous monitoring, i.e. keeping the patient under keen observation.
- In case of greater blood loss, patient should be immediately shifted to hospital for blood transfusion.
- In anaphylactic shock, adrenaline drug should be given, use of corticosteroids is also recommended.

Q 8. Define wound. What are types of wound? Give the first aid treatment for wounds.

Wound

A wound is any breach in the continuity of the skin or mucous membrane which arise from injury.

Types of Wounds

- *Incised wounds*: These are sharp cuts caused by sharp weapons like knife or sword.
- *Lacerated wound*: These are caused by blunt objects such as hammer, stone, etc.

  These wounds have irregular margins and are associated with the damage of the surrounding tissue.
- *Punctured wounds*: These wounds are caused by penetration of pointed and sharp weapons as a pointed knife or screw driver in the body. These wounds may damage internal organs, if these are deep wounds.

Abrasion

These are superficial injuries caused by rubbing or scrapping.

First Aid Treatment of Wounds

- Clean the wound with sterile normal saline solution.
- Cover the wound by applying dressings.
- For bleeding wound, apply firm pressure over the wound after covering it with sterile dressing.

- Dressing should be sterile and dry or soaked in antiseptic solution.
- Bandage or adhesive tape/plaster is used to keep dressings in proper place.
  i. Common antiseptic solutions used are:
     – Acriflavine lotion (AF lotion)

Acriflavine	200 mg
Spirit	75 ml
Sterile water	100 ml

  ii. A gauze piece soaked in this solution are applied over the wounds.
     – Eusol (Edinburgh university solution)

Bleaching powder	1.25 gm
Boric acid	1.25 gm
Calcium hydroxide	1.25 gm
Sterile water	1000 ml

Q 9. What is fracture? What are general signs and symptoms of fracture? What are types of fractures? Give first aid treatment for fracture. (S. 97, 99, 00, 04, 05, 09; W. 97, 00, 03, 04, 05, 07)

Fracture

A fracture is defined as a broken bone or cracked bone.

Signs and Symptoms of Fracture

- Immediate swelling at the affected area.
- Severe pains near the site of fracture.
- Tenderness or discomfort over the affected area on pressure.
- Deformity in bones.
- Dislocation of bones.

Types of Fractures

- *Closed fracture*: A bone is broken beneath the skin but without injury to skin.
- *Compound fractures*: A bone is broken and there is wound leading down to the fracture. In some cases fractured bone may protrude out through such wounds.
- *Complicated fractures*: A fracture with injury to a vessel or nerve or a vital organ.

General First Aid Treatment of Fractures

- Do not move fractured part unless required.
- If bleeding wound is observed, cover it with sterile dressing and also to stop bleeding.
- When a fracture is suspected, do not give anything to the victim by mouth.
- If the victim is suffering from shock, the first aid treatment for shock may be given.
- Take the victim to the hospital as early as possible.

Special Treatment is Necessary for following Fractures

- *For skull fracture*: In an accident a severe blow to head may cause skull fracture.
  i. *Signs and symptoms*
     – Unconscious
     – Bleeding from nose, mouth, ears
     – Paralysis of head muscles including eyelids and tongue.
  ii. *Treatment*
     – Do not move the victim unless necessary.
     – If face colour is reddening, then raise the head and shoulder slightly.
     – If the face colour is pale, then elevate the legs and trunk above the level of head.
     – Loosen the clothing around the neck, chest and trunk.
     – If scalp is bleeding, apply sterile dressing with moderate pressure.
     – Do not give anything by mouth.
     – Give artificial respiration if needed.
- *Neck and spine fractures*
  i. *Signs and symptoms*
     – Severe pains in neck and back region.
     – Paralysis of body parts below the injury spot.
  ii. *Treatment*
     – Do not move the victim until absolutely necessary.
     – If the victim is to be moved, use firm support for moving the victim.
     – Take care that victims head and spine remains on a line.
     – Do not allow victim to rotate the head.
     – Arrange for moving the victim to hospital.

Q 10. What is sunstroke? Give the first aid treatment for sunstroke.

Sunstroke

Sunstroke is an injury caused by extreme heat.

- Sunstroke occurs commonly in elder persons and in those, when head is more exposed to the sun heat.
- Person who wear a hot and cool clothing and also consume a plenty of water may not suffer from sunstroke problem.
- Person suffering from excessive sweating, may produce loss of chlorides that needs salt intake to compensate balance.

Treatments

- Take the victim to the indoor immediately.
- Remove the clothing and go for cooling the body surface by cold water sponging.
- If the victim is conscious, give the victim plenty of water with some salt solution (table salt).
- Try to arrange for transfer of victim to the hospital at the earliest.

Q 11. What are splints? What are different types of splints? (S. 01; W. 98, 00)

Splints

Splints are the rigid materials used to fix the ends of fractured bones and to make it immobile as nearly as possible.

They are made-up of wooden plank, a metal or cardboard, etc.

Types of Splints

- Knee splint.
- Clavicular cross splint.
- Plaster splint.
- Taylor splint.
- Knee splint with protractor.

Q 12. Explain in short the elements of minor surgery and dressing. (S. 06; W. 98, 99, 00)

Elements of minor surgery and dressing means necessary parts of components required for minor operations: These are:

i. Sterile absorbent cotton
ii. Adhesive tape

iii. Dressing bandages
iv. Scissors
v. Forceps
vi. Sponge holding forceps
vii. Sutured surgical needle
viii. Needle holder
ix. Rubber hand gloves
x. Antiseptic cream, e.g. nitrofurazone cream, cetrimide cream.
xi. Local anesthetics, e.g. xylocaine.

Q 13. What is poisoning? Enlist various route by which poisoning may occur. What are general preventive measures to avoid poisoning incidence?

Poisoning

Poisoning is defined as entry of the poisonous substance in the body of individual or upon the surface of body of individual.

Poison

Poisons are the substances which produce harmful or toxic effects on human body.

Routes of Poisoning

- *Oral route*: Contaminated food and water, insecticide, pesticides, alcohol, strong acids and alkalies, narcotics, cause poisoning by oral route.
- *Inhalation*: Inhalation of carbon monoxide, dense smoke from fire, fumes of poisonous chemicals causes poisoning.
- *Injection*: Injection of narcotics, hypnotics, etc.
- *Skin poison or contract poison*: Pesticides, BHC, irritant chemicals, etc.
- *Bites*: As a bite of dog, cat, snakes, bees, etc.

General Preventive Measures to Avoid Poisoning Incidence

- Discard expired medicines immediately by frequent checking of the expiry date.
- Always keep the medicines in light so that information from wrapper can be seen properly and easily.
- Keep the poisonous chemicals always in well-labelled containers and out of reach of hands of children.

- Destroy empty containers very properly and immediately to avoid the misuse.
- Avoid burning of coal or wood or any such fuel material that can produce smoke within closed rooms.
- Examine frequently poisonous plant from surrounding and remove them immediately.
- Cover the food material very properly so that poisoning due to contamination of food can be avoided.

Q 14. Describe the first aid treatment to poisoning.

- If the person is conscious, the vomiting is induced by giving emetics such as syrup of ipecac or salt solution, etc.
- Collect and preserve the vomiting materials which can give some clues about the types of poison used.
- If a person is unconscious or suspected to have consumed acid or strong alkali, do not induce vomiting.
- If the ingested poison is available in stomach, it should be diluted by milk or water.
- If the poisoning has caused interference in breathing, try for artificial respiration.
- If the symptoms are serious, call the doctor immediately and arrange for quick transfer to hospital.
- Try to locate the cause of poisoning by collecting all the information from surrounding and inform the doctor.
- Poisoning is a serious matter and in most cases police has to be informed.

Q 15. Explain general treatments for poisoning. (S. 95; W. 97)

The treatment of a poisoning case consist of following steps:

i. Removal of unabsorbed poison from the body.
ii. Administration of antidote.
iii. Elimination of poison by excretion.
iv. Symptomatic treatment.

1. Removal of Unabsorbed Poison from the Body

- In cases of gas poisoning the patient must be shifted to the open area so that clean and fresh air is made available. This helps to remove gaseous poison. Victims rooms should be ventilated by opening doors and windows.

- If poison is applied locally, i.e. on body surface, it should be washed and rewashed by plain water.
- In conscious patient vomiting is induced
- In unconscious patients stomach wash or gastric levage should be done with the help of stomach tube.

2. Administration of Specific Antidote

Antidote is a substance which stops the action of poison. Specific antidotes for particular case of poisoning are:

- Arsenic poisoning—BAL (Dimercaprol).
- Lead poisoning—EDTA (Ethylenediamine-tetraacetic).
- Opium poisoning—Naloxone hydrochloride.

When type of poison is not known exactly, then (GA) general antidote called as universal antidote can be used.

- Composition of universal antidote
  - i. Magnesium oxide 1 part
  - ii. Tannic oxide 2 parts
  - iii. Activated charcoal 2 parts
  - iv. A glass of warm water

Above mixture is given as oral drink to the victim

3. Elimination of Absorbed Poison

By excretion/or defecation.

- Diuretics such as mannitol increases urination thus helps to excrete the poison.
- Acidic drugs are excreted in alkaline urine and basic drugs are excreted in acidic urine. Thus to excrete the poison nature of urine is change.

4. Symptomatic Treatment

- Maintenance of respiration.
- Cardiac massage.
- To provide energy intravenous glucose saline is given.
- Oxygen inhalation is provided.
- Prevention of secondary infections by use of specific antibiotics.

Q 16. Name the antidotes for various poisoning.

Common Poisons and their Specific Antidotes

S. No.	*Name of the poisons*	*Recommended antidotes*	*Types of the antidotes*
1.	Arsenic bismuth mercury copper, gold and other heavy metals	BAL (Dimercaprol)	Physiological
2.	Lead, mercury, copper cobalt, cadmium, iron and nickel	EDTA (Ethylenediamine-tetraacetic acid)	Chelating agent
3.	Heavy metals	Penicillamine	Chelating agent of maximum efficiency
4.	Iron	Desferrioxamine	Chelating agent
5.	Organophosphorus compounds	DAM (Diacetyl monoxime) atropine sulfate	Cholinesterase reactivators receptor blockers
6.	Opium	Naloxone hydrochloride	Competitive antagonist
7.	Cocaine	Amylnitrate	Dilator of blood vessels
8.	Digitalis	Lignocaine	Antiarrhythmic drug

CHAPTER 5

Environment and Health

Q 1. What is water pollution? Give the causes sources and control measures of water pollution. (S. 95)

Water Pollution

"Pollution of water caused by domestic sewage, toxic chemicals and industrial wastes is called water pollution."

Sources/Causes of Water Pollution

- Domestic wastes may contaminate the water.
- Sewage containing human excreta, urine and dung are discharged into water forms a major source of water pollution.
- Industrial wastes which contain toxic chemicals may pollute water.
- Agricultural wastes like fertilizers, pesticides cause water pollution.
- Thermal waste from thermal and nuclear power plants may discharge large amount of high temperature water into river which may affect aquatic life.
- Radioactive dust formed during atomic explosion contains radioisotopes which get into water and pollute the water.
- Many oil carrying ships moving in the large oceans may meet with an accidents leading to spilling of million of tons of oil in the sea cause water poilution.

Control of Water Pollution

- Educating the people to prevent the pollutants being released into drinking water supply.
- Whenever possible, the drinking water should be provided through the piped water supply.
- Sanitary wells should be provided where the piped water supply is not possible.

- Sewage must be treated both physically, chemically and biologically and then released in the rivers.
- Industrial effluent should be treated to neutralize toxic chemicals and released in the river.
- Water pollutants can be removed by adsorption, electrolysis filtration, etc.
- Prevention and control of water pollution Act was passed in India in 1974 which would ensure legal actions against water polluting bodies.
- Recycling of waste: Dung and urine of cattle can be conveniently used to generate biogas for cooking and heating, etc.

Q 2. Discuss the hazards of water pollution. OR How water pollution affects community? OR What are the effects of water pollution on human health? (S. 97, 99, 00, 01, 03, 05; W. 98)

- Polluted water may cause epidemic disease like cholera, dysentery, typhoid, jaundice, etc.
- Mercury is one of the most toxic metal produces abdominal and chest pains, diarrhoea, mercury poisoning.
- Lead metal cause symptoms like constipation, loss of appetite.
- Arsenic present in the polluted water may cause mental disturbance, liver cirrhosis, lung cancer, kidney damage, etc.
- The insecticides which get accumulated in the body of fish, enters in human body through food chain may cause cancer.
- Deficient O_2 in water due to industrial wastes, kills, fishes and other aquatic animals.

Q 3. What is air pollution? Give the composition of pure air. Mention the functions of pure air.

Air Pollution

"An undesirable changes occurring in air causing harmful effects on man and domestic species is called as Air pollution."

Composition of Pure Air **(S. 95, 96, 97, 98, 02, 03, 05; W. 96, 97, 98, 02)**

i. Oxygen	20.95%
ii. Carbon dioxide	0.03 to 0.4%
iii. Nitrogen	79%
iv. Water vapours	Variable

v. Ammonia
vi. Organic mater
vii. Ozone
viii. Mineral salts

} Traces

Functions of Pure Air

- Pure air is necessary for interchange of gases in the process of respiration.
- The regulation of body temperature.
- Purification of blood.

Q 4. What are the causes and control measures of air pollution? (S. 96, 97, 98, 02, 03, 09; W. 96, 97, 98, 02, 06, 08)

Sources/Causes of Air Pollution

- *Respiration of men and animals*: The major impurities in expired air are CO_2 (4.41%), water vapours and organic matter. In the overcrowding rooms the air becomes stuffy with reduced O_2 content hence may cause symptoms like headache, nausea. During coughing, sneezing and loud speaking by infected patient may leads to air pollution.
- *By combustion*: Burning of coals, oils, lamps may produce smoke may consist of poisonous gases. Domestic smoke sticks to the particles on which they fall and hence produce harmful effects.
- *Industrialization and vehicles*: May industries may produce smoke which pollutes the air. The air pollution may become more severe with more fires, furnaces, more motors and cars, etc.
- *Decomposition*: Animals and vegetables after decomposition gives off poisonous gases like CO_2, H_2S, ammonia which may pollute air.
- *Dust*: The particles in air of houses, contains particles arising from wear and tear of articles may pollute the air, ashes, fibres of cotton, particles of hair spore, pollen grains may pollute the air.

Preventive/Control Measures of Air Pollution

- Health education of the public about harmful effects of air pollution.
- Modification of industrial processes to minimize air pollution by toxic materials.
- Traffic management to reduce pollution.
- Establishment of “green belt” between industrial and residential areas.

- Minimise the use of wood, coal oil, and to promote the use of electricity and natural gas.
- Legal measures to control emission of smoke and other pollutants.
- Disinfection of polluted air can be done by mechanical ventilation, UV radiation, dust control measures, etc.
- Use of high quality fuel in automobiles.
- Use of battery operated vehicles.
- The industrial smoke must be filtered before releasing into the atmosphere.

Q 5. What are problems/hazards/ill effects of air pollution? OR What are the effects of air pollution on human health? (W. 07)

- Allergic diseases like bronchial asthma, bronchitis, and other lung disorders.
- Inhalation of polluted air causes heaviness, sleepiness, headache, vomiting.
- High levels of CO_2 can impair the normal vision of a person.
- CO_2 and nitrous oxide may reduce ability of blood to carry O_2.
- The heavy metal particulate pollutants causes cancer, hypertension, etc.
- SO_2 is a gaseous pollutant and causes drying of mouth.
- Particulate matter such as ash, dust, soot, smoke, etc. causes problems mainly with respiratory tract like irritation, coughing, allergic conditions, etc.
- Over a chronic period, exposure of air pollution leads to conjunctivitis, dermatitis, chronic bronchitis, rickets.

Q 6. What are the "immediate effects" and "delayed effects" of air pollution on human health? (S. 96)

The effects of air pollution on health may be categorised as:

Immediate Effects

It includes adverse effects on functions of respiratory system, e.g. bronchial asthma, irritation, coughing, bronchitis, lung disorders.

Delayed Effects

Over a chronic period exposure, air pollution leads to:

i. Conjunctivitis
ii. Dermatitis
iii. Chronic bronchitis

iv. Pneumoconiosis
v. Rickets
vi. Primary lung cancer.

Q 7. What is noise? What are the sources of noise? What are auditory and nonauditory effects of noise? Give preventive measures to control noise pollution. (S. 95, 96, 99, 00; W, 98, 99, 00, 02, 03, 04, 05)

Noise

Noise is an "unwanted or unaccepted" sound.

- A sound becomes noise when it causes disturbances to the hearer.
- Noise is measured in units of decibel.
- Peoples can tolerate the sound about 85 decibels.
- The sound begins to be uncomfortably loud at an intensity of 100 decibels and painful at 130 to 140 decibels.

Auditory Effects of Noise

- Permanent or temporary deafness.
- Auditory fatigue.
- Tinnitus.
- Damage of internal ear.
- Headache.

Nonauditory Effects of Noise

- Mental abnormality or confusion.
- Rise in blood pressure.
- Increased intracranial tension, heart rate, respiratory rate, etc.
- Increased sweating.
- Nausea, fatigue.
- Insomnia.
- Visual disturbances.

Sources of Noise

Automobiles, factories, industries, aircrafts, domestic noises from radio, television, transistor, atom bombs, etc.

Preventive and Control Measures of Noise

- To educate the public in general about bad effects of noise.
- Promoting interest of the industrial enterprises and transport authorities to control the noise.

- Vehicles must be periodically checked.
- Workers who are exposed to loud noise should be protected by wearing ear protectors or helmets.
- Legislation control.
- Periodic examination of workers is also necessary.
- Avoid the use of noisy machines.

Q 8. What are the ill-effects of sunlight? State various methods to control them. (S. 98)

Ill-effects of Sunlight

- Eye strain.
- Skin-darkening.
- Skin burn/sunstroke.
- Skin cancer.
- Headache.
- Tiredness and loss of efficiency.

Methods to Control Sunlight Effects

- Use sun goggles for the protection of eyes from UV rays.
- Wear hand gloves, hats, etc.
- Use sun-screen lotion and ointment before going into the sunlight, which protects the skin.
- Light coloured walls of the rooms are ideal for good lighting and controlling them.
- To control the excess sunlight ray in the rooms, goggle glasses may be used for windows.

Q 9. Elaborate the adverse effects of poorlight on health. (S. 95)

- Headache.
- Eye strain.
- Tendency to postural deformity.
- Poking head.
- Lateral deviation of spine.
- Irritability of temper.
- Greater liability to accidents.
- Miner's nystagmus is caused by eye strains due to poor light.

Q 10. What are different sources of water supply? Write a note on sources of water supply. (S. 96, 98, 99, 01, 02, 03, 05, 09; W. 96, 97, 02, 05, 07)

The main sources of water supply are:

- Rain water and artificial lakes.
- Surface water, e.g. canals, rivers, tanks, ponds.
- Upland surface water, e.g. lakes.
- Ground water, e.g. wells and springs.
- Sea water.

a. Rain Water

Rain is the primary source of all water. Rain water is pure initially but after coming into atmosphere it becomes impure.

Advantages

- Normal rain water is nonpathogenic.
- It is soft water as it contain no mineral salts.
- Rain water if properly collected and stored, is a safe water.

Disadvantages

- It is soft and liable to corrode lead pipes and cause lead poisoning.
- The impurities such as dust microbes, gases may involved in it from atmosphere. Hence it may cause infection.
- Filtration and sterilization is essential.

b. Surface Water

Rain water on reaching the ground comes to a river, canal, stream, lake or pond and is called surface water.

Advantages

- It can be collected in large reservoir or setting tanks.
- After filtration, sterilization by chlorination it is suitable for drinking.

Disadvantages

- Surface water may contains suspended particles and disease causing agents and thus dangerous to drink.
- It should be filtrated and sterilized before use.

c. Upland Surface Water

Upland surface water runs on the side of hills, slopes and valleys and is taken off as water supply before it forms big streams and rivers.

Advantage

It is safe because it is pure rain water which has travelled a short distance.

Disadvantage

It needs purification by filtration and sterilization by chlorination.

d. Ground Water

Ground water is superior to surface water. Wells and springs are important sources of ground water. An ideal well should be tapped in a good soil and should be at least 200 feets away from possible contamination source.

Advantages

- It is of good quality.
- No contamination of water on keeping long storage.
- It is free from pathogens.
- Usually requires no treatment.

Disadvantages

- High mineral content.
- Require lifting arrangement to water.
- The usual ground water source of wells and springs.

e. Sea water

Sea water is last and very large reservoir of water. The water from river, canals, stream is finally collected in the sea water. It may contain dust particles, pathogenic organisms, gases, salts, etc.

Advantages

It is a large reservoir.

Disadvantages

- Nonsuitable for drinking as such: Purification and treatment is necessary to use water for drinking purpose.

Q 11. What are different methods of "purification of water"? (W. 04)

Methods of purification of water

On small scale

a. Boiling
b. By using chemicals such as bleaching powder, $KMnO_4$
c. Filtration

On large scale

a. Storage
b. Chlorination
c. Filtration
   - → Slow sand filters
   - → Rapid sand filters

Q 12. Describe the design and mechanism of septic tank. (S. 99, 09; W. 99, 00, 01, 06, 08)

- Septic tank is a sewage settling tank is which household waste water and excreta can be disposed off.
- As the sewage enters the tank, sedimentation occurs from the upper portion.
- A septic tank should have a minimum capacity of 2,00,000 litres.
- It is not suitable for very big communities.
- Septic tank is rectangular on the surface.
- Water is filled in the septic tanks, height of water column is 1 to 1.5 metres.
- There is an inlet and outlet pipe above the water level and air space above the water level.
- A cover of cement concrete is provided at the top with manhole in the center and the manhole is covered with another lid.

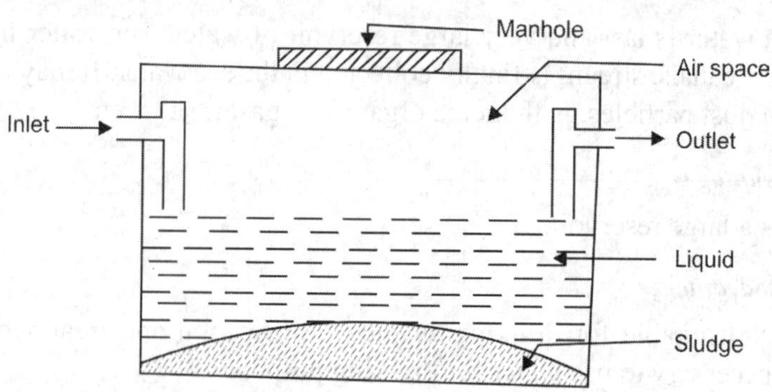

Mechanism

- The mechanism of septic tank is anaerobic digestion of the contents.
- The heavy solids settles down and decomposed by anaerobic bacteria which causes reduction it its volume and is rendered harmless.
- The solid at the bottom is called "sludge".
- The fatty and greasy substance rise to the water surface above and is passed out through the outlet pipe.
- Since this supernatant liquid effluent contains microorganisms, ova, it is allowed to be collected in trenches.
- It spreads in the soil, microorganisms die out and organic matter gets oxidised. This stage is called aerobic decomposition.
- The sludge from the bottom is removed every year as more sludge interferes with the working of the tank.
- This sludge is buried in trenches.

Q 13. Discuss the methods used for purification of water on small scale. (S. 95, 98, 01, 03; W. 96, 01)

There are three methods used for purifying water on small scale a. Boiling, b. Chemical disinfection, c. Filtration.

a. Boiling

Boiling water for 10 minutes kills all living microorganisms and their spores and water becomes sterile. Some of the salts present in water are also precipitated and hence there is a little change in taste also, i.e. it also removes temporary hardness of water. Water should be boiled preferably in same container, in which it is to be stored to avoid contamination during storage.

b. Chemical Disinfection (S. 04)

By using following chemicals.

i. *Bleaching powder or chlorinated lime*: A fresh sample of bleaching powder contains 33% chlorine and if chlorine is 25% it is acceptable for disinfection of water. To make bleaching powder more stable, lime is added to it and such sample is called stabilized bleach.

Bleaching powder is stored in dry, cool and dark places in air tight container. Amount of bleaching powder needed for one cubic metre water is 2.3 gm which leaves 0.5 mg chlorine/litre of water after one hour contact.

ii. *Chlorine tablets*: These are small tablets available for various quantities of water to be disinfected. They are comparatively stable and one tablet of 0.5 gm is sufficient for 20 litres of water.
iii. *Iodine*: 2% alcoholic solution of iodine can disinfect 1 litre of water within ½ an hour. It is used only in emergencies because it may give rise to thyroid disorders.
iv. *Potassium permanganate*: It is strong oxidizing agent and can kill cholera bacteria. It alters the taste, smell and colour of water.

c. Filtration

Small household filters are available. The filtering is done either through porcelain material or earth. Filters do not filter the viruses as they are very small in size. The filters are regularly washed with scrubbing to keep them in good condition. Only clear water is used in filters.

Q 14. Describe the methods used for purification of water on large scale. (S. 96, 00, 01; W. 96, 98, 00, 08)

On large scale water is purified in three stages: a. Storage, b. filtration, c. chlorination.

a. Storage

It allows natural purification of water. The water is stored in large reservoirs. Almost all suspended particles settle down at the bottom and water becomes transparent and the action of natural sunlight is better on water. The organic matter present in water is oxidised by bacteria with the help of dissolved oxygen present in water. The water should not be stored for more than 2 weeks as algae and other aquatic vegetation grow on prolonged storage which may give bad colour and taste.

b. Filtration

This is the next stage of purification of water after storage and this removes almost 98–99% bacteria. Two types of filters used are:

i. Slow sand filters (biological filters).
ii. Rapid sand filters (mechanical filters).

c. Chlorination

It is most important and the last stage in water purification. It is supplement to the storage and filtration. On large scale, chlorination is done by bleaching powder. The sample should contain at least 25% chlorine. Chlorine kill the bacteria, oxidizes organic matter and to some extent it can remove bad taste and smell. The chemical reaction of water and chlorine is:

$$H_2O + Cl_2 \longrightarrow HCl + HOCl$$
$$HOCl \longrightarrow [H] + [OCl]$$

HCl is hydrochloric acid which is neutralized by the alkalinity of water. HOCl is hypochlorous acid which further breaks down into hydrogen and hypochlorite ions (OCl). The bactericidal action because of hypochlorous acid (HOCl) and hypochlorite ion (OCl). Hypochlorous acid acts best in neutral pH, i.e. 7.

Chlorination is effective only if water is clear. The need of chlorine is estimated, i.e. now much chlorine will disinfect water, which is called "chlorine demand" of water. When processes of disinfection is complete, free chlorine starts appearing in water. The point, where free chlorine appears in water is called "breaking point". The time for which chlorine is allowed to act in water is called "contact period", which is at least 1 hour. To avoid contamination in future during water transportation and storage, some free chlorine is left in water.

Q 15. What is sewage? What are the aims of sewage purification? Elaborate biological treatment of sewage. How disposal of sewage is done? Write a note on sewage. (S. 96, 97, 05; W. 96, 98, 00, 05, 06, 07)

Sewage

Sewage is polluted material contain waste water, excreta, industrial waste and waste water from public places. Sewage looks like very dirty water with a bad smell. Sewage is a water contains 0.1% solids. The solids includes organic and inorganic substances, microorganisms, dust, fibres. The organic matter partly decomposes naturally during the passage by the action of bacteria, present in it and thus it is foul smelling.

Sewage Treatment

In modern sewage plants certain biological and chemical changes takes place. The processes are aerobic and anaerobic decomposition of the organic matter by bacteria present in it. The big solid particles are removed by screening and sedimentation. Sewage treatment involves two stages:

i. *Primary treatment*: It includes the removal of big solid objects and sedimentation associated with anaerobic respiration. It is carried out in two different steps:

a. *Screening*: The sewage from public sewers is passed through a special screen to remove floating wood, dead animals or any other big objects.
b. *Grit settling chamber*: The screened sewage is allowed to pass through a long chamber of 10–12 metres in length slowly so that heavy particles like sand, small stones, grit, etc. settle down at the bottom. The settled material is removed from the chamber and disposed of by burying. Primary sedimentation tank is used for this purpose to separate "effluents" and "sludge". Effluents undergoes secondary treatment.

ii. *Secondary treatment*: Effluents are treated with the antimicrobial agents to kill all the microbes and then they are passed to the rivers.

Q 16. What are solid wastes/refuse? What are the sources of solid wastes? What are the hazards of accumulated solid waste? Describe the methods of disposal of solid wastes/refuse. (S. 95, 97, 01, 04, 05, 07, 08, 09; W. 96, 97, 99, 00, 03, 07)

Solid Wastes/Refuse

"Solid waste or refuse is the unwanted waste material from the industries, houses, streets and agricultural activities."

Refuse is harmful to human health because when it decomposes and ferments, it attracts flies, rodents, pigs and other animals. Therefore, refuse should be collected in a sanitary manner, transported and disposed of as quickly as possible.

Sources of Refuse

- Street refuse collected by cleaning street.
- Market refuse, e.g. rotten fruits and vegetables, leaves, animals droppings.
- Industrial refuse.
- The domestic refuse, e.g. ashes, paper, metal wood, glass, dust, garbage.

Hazards of Solid Waste Accumulation

- Fermentation of organic matter gives bad odour and may helps in fly breeding.
- Refuse attracts rats, flies which convey pathogens to man.
- There is a risk of air pollution.

- There is a possibility of water pollution if rain water passes through deposits of fermenting refuse.

Disposal of Solid Wastes/Refuse

The principle methods of refuse disposal are:

- Dumping.
- Manure pits.
- Burning.
- Sanitary land filling.
- Composition.
- Burial.

a. Dumping

The refuse is dumped in low areas and pits and the surface is made level and is suitable only for dry refuse. It is not preferred nowadays because it causes public nuisance, attracts insects and animals and causes air and water pollution.

b. Manure Pits

They can be used at household level. Every house should have a manure pits and refuse of all types from the house should be put into it and covered by earth in the evening. When pits is full it is covered with earth and left for 6 months. It gives manures for field.

c. Burning

- It is also called incineration.
- It is suitable for hospital refuse.
- It requires sufficient space and a special equipment called as "incinerator".
- It is a hollow cylinder made up of metal.
- The refuse is put on the land and covered with incinerator before burning to avoid spread during burning.
- In India it is not suitable because it is a direct loss of manure and the process is expensive.

d. Sanitary Land Filling

- A trench is dug.
- The refuse is put in the trench and covered with earth everyday.
- When the trench is nearby full it is covered with earth and is impacted.
- Sometimes alternate layer of refuse and mud are replaced in the trench till it is full.

- Once trench is full it is covered.
- Due to chemical and bacteriological process, decompose the refuse into simple substances with generation of heat.
- The temperature rises over 60°C within a week and cools down in 15 to 20 days.
- The refuse is fully decomposed at the end of 6 months and can be used as manure.

e. Compositing

- In this method refuse and excreta is disposed of together.
- The basic principle is that when the refuse and excreta are dumped in a pit and covered with earth there is anaerobic decomposition and disease producing organisms also die because of heat and ultimately we get "compost" which is used as manure.

f. Burial

In this method small trench is dug and refuse is put in and covered with earth everyday, when full it is covered with earth and another trench is dug.

Q 17. Explain the method of excreta disposal. Discuss the important features of RCA latrine.

RCA Latrine

It is a most accepted type is designed by Research cum action (RCA) project, government of India.

Important Features of RCA Latrine

Location

A dug well is needed for RCA latrine, to avoid all possibilities of ground water contamination a distance of minimum 15 metres should be kept from any source of water.

Features of RCA Latrine

- *Squatting plate*: It is called squatting plate because Indians use squatting posture for defecation. It should have a square stage of minimum 90 cm × 90 cm lined with cement and should have slight slope towards the centre to facilitate cleaning. Raised foot rest may be provided for comfort.

- *Pan*: It is the receptacle of faecal matter, urine and wash water. It is broad at back and narrow at the front end. The length from front to back is 42.5 cm, the width of widest portion is 20 cm and narrowest portion is 12.5 cm. The pan is having smooth, uniform and pervious finish and a hole is provided at the back end.
- *Trap*: It is a bent pipe of 7.5 cm diameter. Its vertical portion is attached with pan. It holds some water and water level is called water seal. It is usually 2 cm.
- *Connecting pipe*: The bend end of the trap is attached with the connecting pipe of the same diameter 7.5 cm for carrying the faeces to dug well.

The dug well has 75 cm diameter and 3–4 metre in depth.

Sometimes a latrine without a connecting pipe is constructed and dug well is just below the installation. This is called direct RCA latrine. Latrine with the connecting pipe is called indirect RCA latrine.

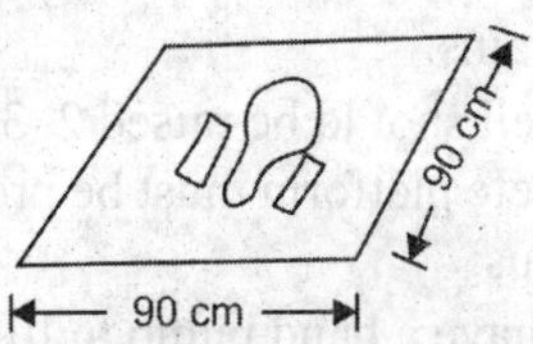

(a) Squatting plate

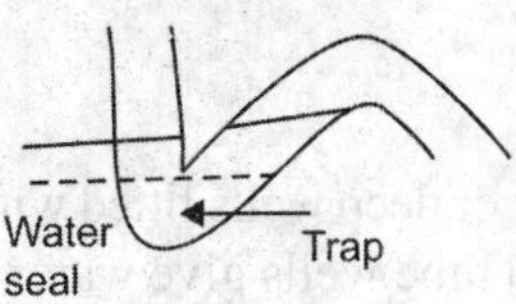

(b) Trap

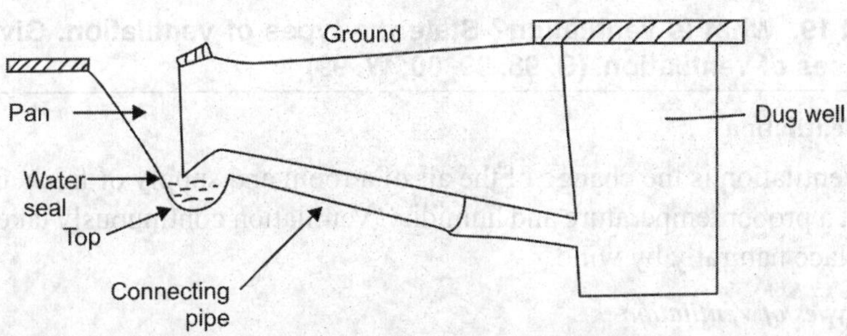

(c) Indirect RCA latrine squatting plate

Q 18. What are different types of wells?

Wells have been classified into: Shallow wells, sanitary wells, tube wells, dug wells.

a. Shallow Wells

Shallow well is one which provides water from the first impervious layer of ground and deep well taps water from below the first impervious layer.

b. Sanitary Wells

Features

- All the *kaccha* wells should be made *pacca* by providing an impervious lining at least up to 20 feet depth.
- The location of well should not be very near to living places and not very far off. The distance should be 15 to 100 metres.
- The well should be elevated from the ground to minimise contamination during rains.
- The lining of the well should be raised 2–3 feet above the ground and a cement concrete platform must be provided around the well within 1 metre radius.
- Every well should have a hand pump to lift the water.
- Safety and potability of sanitary well water depends on behaviour of user community.

c. Tube Wells

They are also shallow or deep wells fitted with pumping arrangement, the hand pump. Deep tube wells give water throughout the year and do not depend upon rain fall.

Q 19. What is ventilation? State the types of ventilation. Give uses of ventilation. (S. 98, 99, 00; W. 99)

Ventilation

Ventilation is the change of the air of a room and supply of fresh air at a proper temperature and humidity. Ventilation continuously takes place naturally by wind.

Types of Ventilation

- Ventilation provided in the form of a window.

- Cross ventilation: It means when the windows and doors are facing each other and if winds blows from one it can easily pass through the other.
- Ventilation by efficient exhaust system.
- Mechanical ventilation by fan, electric devices.

Uses of Ventilation

- Ventilation keeps pure air in the houses.
- Ventilation by natural wind always exchanges the air in the houses.
- Ventilation is the requirement of first aid proper treatment for some of the patients.

CHAPTER 6

Fundamental Principles of Microbiology

Q 1. Define the terms microbiology and 'microorganism'. Classify microorganisms. (S. 96, 98, 99, 01, 02, 04, 07, 09; W. 96, 97, 98, 05, 07)

Microbiology

Microbiology is the branch of science which deals with the study of identification, structure, physiology, metabolism and reproduction of microorganisms.

Microorganisms

Microorganisms are a heterogeneous group of several distinct classes of living beings.

Classification

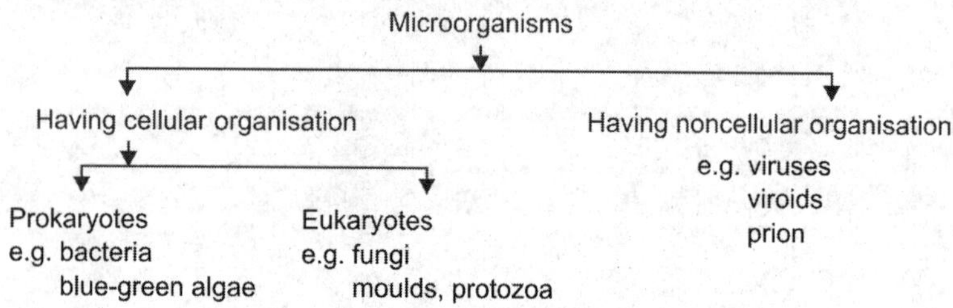

Q 2. Define and classify viruses with examples. Enlist living and nonliving characters of viruses. (S. 97, 98, 01; W. 01)

Viruses

Viruses are noncellular, ultramicroscopic highly infectious agent and posses only one type of nucleic acid.

Classification

Viruses

- DNA viruses (They contains DNA) e.g. herpes virus, pox virus
- RNA viruses (They contains RNA) e.g. measles virus, rabies virus

Living characters of virus	Nonliving characters of virus
i. They posses nucleic acid and proteins.	i. They do not show cellular organisation.
ii. They are capable of reproduction.	ii. They carry out their own metabolic activities.
iii. They transmit hereditary characters from generation to generation.	iii. They are inactive outside a host cell.
iv. They are sensitive to chemicals, heat and UV rays.	iv. They possess either DNA or RNA.
v. They are capable undergoing mutations.	v. They can be crystallized like other nonliving chemical substances.

Q 3. What are stains and dyes? What is the purpose of staining? What are the types of staining? (S. 99, 00, 01, 05, 06, 07; W. 97)

Stain

Stains are the organic dyes used for staining the microorganisms.

Examples

Crystal violet, methylene blue, hematoxylin-eosin, carbolfuschin.

Purpose of Staining

- For greater visualization of cells.
- For study of their structures.
- To differentiate the cells.
- To inhibit the growth of some organism so the others can be visualized.

Types of staining

- A. Simple staining
- B. Differential staining
  - Gram staining
  - Acid-fast staining (Ziehl-Neelsen method)

Q 4. Write a note on gram's staining technique. (S. 00, 04, 08, 09; W. 96, 97, 99, 00, 02, 07, 08)

Christian gram was developed differential staining technique, to differentiate types of bacteria and their specific structure. Hence called as gram's staining.

Gram Staining Procedure

a. Gram-positive Staining

- First the bacteria are taken and carefully spread on a clean glass dry slide. This is called as smear.
- This smear is dried by passing it over a small blue flame. Care should be taken to keep the smear upside.
- Add gention or crystal violet solution and stain is allowed to remain on smear for 30–60 seconds.
- Remove excess stain with water.
- Then add iodine solution for at least 60 seconds.
- Wash with water.
- Finally wash the slide with alcohol or acetone.
- Wash the smear with tap water and observed under microscope.

Observation

If the bacteria have taken up the stain and appears a deep violet or purple black, then they are called as gram-positive bacteria, e.g. staphylococci, streptococci, pneumococci, *E. coli. B. anthracis*, *Clostridium tetani*.

b. *Gram-negative Staining*

- Staining procedure is similar to above.
- If bacteria do not retain crystal violet stain then it is counter stained by safranin for 10 seconds.
- Washed with water and the smear is dried and observed under microscope.

Observation

If bacteria are stained with safranin and pink or red colour is produced. These are called as gram-negative bacteria, e.g. gonococci, meningococci, *E. coli*, *S. typhi*, *H. influenzae*.

Q 5. Write a note on Ziehl-Neelsen's acid fast staining method. (S. 99, 06)

Acid fast microorganisms are:

- *Mycobacterium tuberculosis.*
- *Mycobacterium leprae.*

Ziehl-Neelsen's Staining Procedure

Scientist Ziehl and Neelsen discovered this method. It is important for separation of "Mycobacteria Group" members from others. Ziehl-Neelsen acid fast staining method is most commonly used for a diagnostic aid in identification of species.

Procedure of Staining

- A smear is prepared from the given tubercle sputum and fixed on slide by heat.
- On the smear a Ziehl-Neelsen carbol fuschin stain is added and allowed to react for 10 minutes.
- Precautions were taken to avoid the boiling of stain.
- Wash the smear with water.
- Add 20% H_2SO_4 for one minute and wash it with water.
- Add methylene blue or malachite green for 30 seconds.
- Wash the slide and dry and observe under oil immersion lens.

Observation

- Cells those appears pinkish red are acid fast cells/bacteria.
- Cells those appears blue/green are nonacid fast bacteria.

Q 6. What do you mean by "isolation"? Describe various techniques of isolation of microorganisms. (S. 97, 99, 00, 01, 06, 07, 08; W. 98, 00, 05)

Isolation

Isolation is defined as separating completely and obtaining in pure form of particular type of microorganisms, separating it from its habitat.

Methods of Isolation

- Streak plate method.
- Pour plate method.

- Single cell isolation.
- Direct transfer technique.
- Serial dilution technique.

a. Streak Plate Method **(S. 04)**

- In this method small amount (a loop-full) of sample is transferred on a suitable sterile solid nutrient medium in petridish.
- The sample is streaked by a Nichrome-Wire loop in such a way that, streaking provides successive dilution and thereby the isolated colonies.
- Streaking a solid culture medium in a petridish can be done by following methods.
    i. *Square method:* One loopful suspension is streaked on solid nutrient medium in horizontal line first. Then plate/dish is rotated anticlockwise in 90° and again streaks are made in vertical lines giving rise to square of streaking. The last square will give maximum dilution of sample and so the isolated colonies.
    ii. *Four quadrant method:* A loopful of sample is placed at one spot ½ cm away from periphery of petridish, on solid culture medium. From this, place linear streaks are made. Then from end of first streak second streaks are made by rotating plate anticlockwise. Likewise four streaks are made. Care is taken so that last streaks are made. Care is taken so that last streak do not touch the original spot. On last streak (i.e. on fourth quadrant) maximum. Dilution of sample is achieved and so, on last steak isolated colonies are obtained.
    iii. *Zig-zag method*: A loopful of sample is streaked on solid nutrient agar medium in zig-zag manner. This also allows maximum dilution of terminal end of zig-zag streak, where isolated colonies are obtained.

b. Pour Plate Method

To obtain pure culture by isolation via pour plate method, serial dilutions of the given sample are necessary.

For serial dilution, a set of tubes each containing 9 ml sterile distilled water is taken. Then 10 ml of original sample is added to first tube containing distilled water. From this tube 1 ml is added or transferred to second tube containing 9.0 ml distilled water and so on.

Finally 1 ml of any suitable dilution is mixed with sterilized, melted and cooled nutrient medium in sterile petridish. The contents are mixed thoroughly by gentle rotation of petridish. The contents are then allowed to cool and solidify. Such plates are then incubated for specific time period, to obtained-isolated colonies.

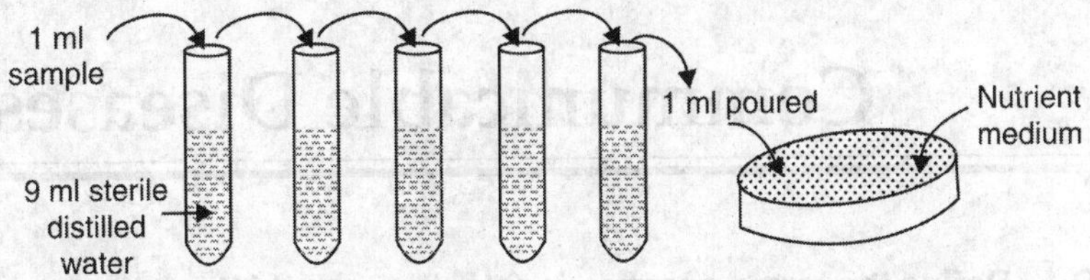

c. Single Cell Isolation by Micromanipulator

- In this method single cell of desired type can be pick out from the mixed culture. This can be done by micromanipulator in combination with microscope.
- Micromanipulator has a micropipette with a very fine capillary point. The micropipette can be moved as desired.
- A single cell can be moved as desired.
- A single cell can be picked by using micropipette and transferred to a suitable nutrient medium.

d. Direct Transfer Technique

Sometimes bacteria, yeast and moulds may be found in pure culture under natural conditions. Such cultures can be directly transferred to a suitable medium and incubated to get number of colonies.

e. Serial Dilution Technique

In this techniques serial dilution of bacteia is done in a series of test tubes.

A small amount of the mixture of bacteria is added to a test tube containing sterile medium of known volume. One ml of liquid bacteia mixture is then diluted to the desired dilution by transfer through a series of test tubes containing similar volume of sterilized medium. A stage will be reached when higher dilutions will contain no organisms and will show no growth upon incubation.

Some of the tubes of higher dilution showing growth will be found to contain only one colony of a species which can be observed by microscopic examination.

CHAPTER 7

Communicable Diseases

Q 1. Define the terms communicable diseases. List out the common communicable diseases prevailing in India. (S. 95, 96, 98, 99, 03; W. 96)

Communicable Diseases

Communicable diseases are defined as an illness due to specific infections agent or its toxic products, capable of being directly or indirectly transmitted from man to man, animal to animal or from environment to man or animal.

The common communicable diseases prevailing in India are:

i. Respiratory infections, e.g. chickenpox, measles, influenza, diphtheria, tuberculosis, whooping cough.
ii. Intestinal infections, e.g. hepatitis, cholera, typhoid, poliomyelitis, food poisoning, hookworm infection.
iii. Arthropod borne infections, e.g. plague, malaria, filaria.
iv. Sexually transmitted diseases, e.g. AIDS, syphilis, gonorrhoea.
v. Surface infections, e.g. rabies, trachoma, leprosy, tetanus.

Q 2. Give the causative agent, mode of transmission, prevention and control of chickenpox. (S. 99, 06; W. 02, 03, 07)

Chickenpox (Varicella)

- *Causative agent*: Chickenpox is an acute highly contagious disease caused by a virus called as varicella-zoster virus (V-Z virus)
- *Incubation period*: 14 to 16 days.
- *Mode of transmission*:
  i. Chickenpox is transmitted from person to person by droplet infection.
  ii. Virus enters the upper respiratory tract commonly.

iii. Sometimes the diseases spreads by contamination from the discharge from ruptured lesions of the skin.

- *Prevention and control*:
  i. Isolation of patient.
  ii. Disinfect all the articles used by the patient.
  iii. Passive immunization by varicella-zoster immunoglobulin given within 72 hours of exposure in the dose of 1.25 to 5 ml by IM injection.
  iv. There is a no specific treatment for chickenpox.

Q 3. Describe the cause mode of transmission, prevention and control of "measles" or "rubeola. (S. 98, 99, 01, 02, 08)

Meascle

It is a highly infectious disease caused by RNA paroxysmal virus of rubella virus.

- *Incubation period:* 10 to 14 days
- *Mode of transmission*
  i. Its spread is direct from person to person through droplet infection, i.e. sneezing, talking, kissing.
  ii. Direct contact with fomite such as spoons, cups and other articles used by the patient.
- *Prevention of measles*
  i. Immunization of measles vaccine.
  ii. Administration of human measles immunoglobulin.
- *Control of meascles*
  i. Isolation of patient.
  ii. Protect the eyes of the patients from light and glare.
  iii. Disinfection of nose and throat discharges.
  iv. Immunise the susceptible children.

Q 4. Name the agent causing tuberculosis. Give the mode of transmission and control measures. (S. 96, 97, 98, 99, 02, 04, 09; W. 98, 99, 00, 02, 03, 05, 06, 07, 08)

Tuberculosis

- *Causative agent*: Tuberculosis is a chronic infections disease caused by *Mycobacterium tuberculosis*.
- *Mode of spread/transmission*
  i. It is transmitted by droplet infection.

ii. By inhaling fine dust particles containing tubercle bacilli.
iii. By direct contact with sputum of infected persons.
iv. By direct contact with the patient.
v. By consuming contaminated foods.

- *Prevention and control*
  i. Early detection of tuberculosis patient by the examination of sputum.
  ii. Isolation of infected patient.
  iii. Use of chemotherapeutic agents like INH, PAS, ethambutol.
  iv. BCG vaccination is used for immunization.
  v. People should be given health education.
  vi. Milk should be consumed after proper boiling.
  vii. The people should be taught about importance of personal hygiene maintaining good sanitation and clean environment, immunization.

Q 5. Name the agent causing "influenza". Describe the mode of transmission, prevention and control of influenza (flue). (S. 99; W. 02, 06)

Influenza

- *Causative agent*: It is an acute infection of respiratory tract caused by influenza viruses A, B, C.
- *Incubation period*: 1 to 2 days.
- *Mode of transmission*
  i. By droplet infection or droplet nuclei created by sneezing coughing and talking.
  ii. By direct contact.
  iii. Through articles recently used by the patient.
- *Prevention*: Use of influenza vaccines.
- *Control*
  i. Early detection and notification to the health authorities.
  ii. Isolate the suspected cases.
  iii. Avoid overcrowding of the places.
  iv. Gargling with normal saline.
  v. Sneezing, spitting, coughing in public places should be avoided.
  vi. The clothes, beddings, fomites and rooms used by the patient should be thoroughly disinfected.
  vii. Used of antiviral drugs like amantadine.

Q 6. Name the agent causing diphtheria. Describe the mode of transmission, prevention and control of diphtheria. (S. 99, 01, 07; W. 01, 02, 03)

Diphtheria

- *Causative agent*: Diphtheria is an acute infectious disease caused by the exotoxin of *Corynebacterium diphtheriae*.
- *Incubation period*: 1 to 2 days.
- *Mode of transmission*
  i. Direct contact
  ii. Droplet infection through coughing and sneezing.
  iii. Indirectly through fomites or contaminated articles such a spoons, cups, toys, etc.
- *Prevention and control of measures*
  i. Early detection and notification to health authorities.
  ii. Isolation of patients.
  iii. Immunization by diphtheria antitoxin.
  iv. All infants should be immunized with DPT (triple vaccine), i.e. diphtheria pertussis and tetanus vaccine.

Q 7. Name the agent causing "whooping cough" or "pertussis". Describe the mode of transmission, prevention and control of whooping cough. (S. 99, 00, 02; W. 97, 06)

Whooping Cough/Pertussis

- *Causative agent*: Whooping cough is an infectious disease of respiratory tract caused by *Bordetella pertussis*.
- *Mode of transmission*
  i. By droplet infection.
  ii. By direct contact when patient talks, sneezes, the bacilli are sprayed into the air.
- *Incubation period*: 7 to 14 days.
- *Prevention control*
  i. Early detection of the disease.
  ii. Isolation of the patients.
  iii. Treatment and disinfection of discharges from nose and throat of patients.
  iv. Cough preparations and antibiotics may be given to the patient.
  v. Every child must be immunised against "whooping cough".

Q 8. Discuss the cause, mode of transmission and prevention of hepatitis A, hepatitis B (serum hepatitis). (S. 97, 98, 01, 03, 08; W. 98, 99, 02, 01, 05)

Hepatitis A

- *Causative agent*: Hepatitis A is an acute infectious disease of liver caused by hepatitis A virus (HAV).
- *Mode of transmission*
  - i. Faecal-oral route: It is spread through contaminated water and food.
  - ii. Direct contact: It can occur directly from person to person or indirectly by using contaminated water, milk, food, etc.
  - iii. Sexual transmission: This may occur mainly among the homosexual men.
- *Incubation period*: 15 to 45 days.
- *Prevention and control*
  - i. Isolation of hepatitis cases.
  - ii. Disinfection of the faeces and fomites and the patient.
  - iii. Anti-fly measures should be taken.
  - iv. Needles and syringes should be properly sterilized.
  - v. Human normal immunoglobulin should be administered to all contacts before or within a week of exposure.
  - vi. Follow personal and community hygienic measures such as washing of hands after toilet and before meals, sanitary disposal of human excreta. Using safe drinking water.

Hepatitis B

- *Causative agent*: Hepatitis B is caused by hepatitis B virus (HBV) which affect the liver.
- *Incubation period*: 60 to 180 days.
- *Mode of transmission*
  - i. Parenteral route: Through infected blood and blood products, dialysis, contaminated needles and syringes.
  - ii. Transmission from HBV carrier mothers to their babies.
  - iii. Transmission by sexual contact or even by kissing.
  - iv. Blood sucking arthropods such as mosquitoes (can transmit the disease.)
- *Prevention and control*
  - i. Avoid blood transfusion and its products which are contaminated with hepatitis B virus.

ii. By the use of sterilised syringes and needles.
iii. Give hepatitis B vaccine by intramuscular route.
iv. Hepatitis B immunoglobulin (HBIg) should be given immediately to the persons who are exposed to hepatitis B virus.
v. Health education.

Q 9. Describe the cause, mode of transmission, prevention and control of typhoid. (S. 95, 99, 02; W. 97, 00, 02, 03, 07, 08)

Typhoid

- *Causative agent*: Typhoid fever is an acute communicable disease caused by *Salmonella typhi*.
- *Incubation period*: 7 to 28 days (average 14 days).
- *Mode of transmission*
  i. Water and food contaminated with faeces or urine of infected person.
  ii. Flies also play a significant role in the spread of this disease.
  iii. Direct contact with infected person.
  iv. Also can be transmitted directly through contaminated hands or fingers with stools of the patients.
- *Prevention and control*
  i. Proper isolation of patients to prevent spreading of disease.
  ii. Water and milk should be consumed only after proper boiling.
  iii. Excreta and urine of infected person should be disposed of in a sanitary way.
  iv. Detection of typhoid carriers and treating them.
  v. Immunization with antityphoid vaccines.
  vi. Antifly measures should be taken.
  vii. Public should be educated for sanitation and personal hygiene.
  viii. Provision of safe drinking water, boiled milk is necessary.
  ix. Public should be immunised with TAB vaccine which contains *S. typhi*, *S. paratyphi* A and *S. paratyphi* B.
  x. Chloramphenicol is the drug of choice for the treatment of typhoid.

Q 10. Name the agent causing cholera. How the disease spreads? Give its prevention and control measures. (S. 95, 02; W. 02)

Cholera

- *Causative agent*: Cholera is caused by an agent *Vibrio cholerae*.
- *Incubation period*: A few hours to 5 days.

- *Mode of transmission*
  i. It spreads by ingestion of contaminated water, food, milk, milk products with discharge of patient.
  ii. By careless handling of excreta and vomites of infected persons.
  iii. Flies can act as mechanical carries.
  iv. Contact with clothes and utensils used by infected persons.
- *Prevention and control of cholera*
  i. Detection of the cases as early as possible and immediately notify to health authorities.
  ii. Isolation of the patient in the hospital or at home.
  iii. Immediately starts Oral Rehydration Therapy (ORS).
  iv. Patients clothes and utensils should be thoroughly disinfect.
  v. Patients stools and vomits should be collected in a pot contaminated some disinfectants and disposed of immediately.
  vi. All latrines and drains, etc. should be cleaned with phenyl or bleeding powder.
  vii. Milk must be boiled before use.
  viii. Antifly measures should be taken.
  ix. All the foods, drinks and sweet meats must be protected against flies.
  x. Special care must be taken regarding the cleanliness of the surrounding as well as personal hygiene.

Q 11. Write a note on food poisoning. (S. 97, 02, 03, 08; W. 97, 98, 00, 06, 08)

Food Poisoning

Food poisoning is an acute gastroenteritis caused by ingestion of food or drink contaminated with either living bacteria or their toxins or chemical substances.

Types of Food Poisoning

i. Chemical food poisoning.
ii. Food poisoning from plants and animals.
iii. Food poisoning by bacteria and their toxins.

- *Chemical food poisoning*: It is caused by ingestion of chemical poisons such as arsenic, cadmium, cyanide, fluorides, fertilizers, pesticides.

- *Food poisoning from plants and animals*: Ingestion of certain varieties of poisonous mushrooms may cause food poisoning.
- *Food poisoning by bacteria and their toxins*: Food poisoning by bacteria and their toxins is the commonest cause of food poisoning which is generally caused by ingestion of food and drinks contaminated with bacteria and their toxins.

  Bacterial food poisoning is of following types:

  i. *Salmonella food poisoning*: It is caused by Salmonella group of microorganisms which includes *S. typhi* and *S. enteritidis*. Foods like milk, milk products, eggs, meat, fish and stored food get contaminated with these bacteria.

  ii. *Staphylococcus food poisonings*: *Staphylococcus aureus* cause poisoning in food which spreads from ice-creams, milk, milk products, cakes, etc.

  iii. *Botulism*: It is a fatal form of food poisoning which is caused by the ingestion of food contaminated with neurotoxins produced by *Clostridium botulinum* which in under-processed, preserved foods, preserved pickles, fruits, vegetables, etc.
- *Prevention and control*

  i. Food should be freshly prepared and eaten at the same time.

  ii. Foods must be protected against flies, rats, mice, and dust.

  iii. Surplus food should be kept in a refrigerator or cool place.

  iv. Personal hygiene and food sanitation should be ensured by the individual particularly engaged in the handling, preparation and cooking of the food.

  v. It should be checked that food animals and meat should be free from any kind of disease.

  vi. Restaurants, hotels and messes or places where food is cooked should be supervised strictly for the quality and hygienic cooking methods.

Q 12. Write a note on botulism. (S. 00, 01)

Botulism is a fatal form of food poisoning which is caused by the ingestion of food contaminated with neurotoxins produced by *Clostridium botulinum* which is found in under-processed, preserved foods, preserved pickles, fruits and vegetables, etc.

- The optimum temperature for growth of this bacteria and for the production of toxins is considered to be 37°C.

- The *Clostridium botulinum* can withstand storage conditions and remain present in precooked frozen foods.
- The symptoms of botulism appear within 12–20 hours after the consumption of food.
- The symptoms includes:
  i. Nausea and vomiting, headache
  ii. Diarrhoea, dryness of mouth
  iii. Double vision
  iv. Decreased salivary secretions
  v. Death may occur in 4–6 days due to heart or respiratory failure.
- *Clostridium botulinum* can withstand moist heat at 100°C for several hours.
- They are destroyed by moist heat at 120°C usually within 5 minutes.

Q 13. Write a note on hookworm infection/infestation. (S. 08)

Hookworm Infection/Infestation/Ancyclostomiasis

- *Causative agent*: Hookworm infection is caused by two types of hookworms *Ancylostoma duodenale* and *Necator americanus*.
- *Mode of transmission*
  i. A single female worm may lay 10,000 to 20,000 eggs per day which are passed in faeces.
  ii. When they happen to be laid on warm moist soil the eggs hatch into larvae (in about 5 days time) where they grow and develop into infective larvae.

  When a person walks bare foot on the contaminated soil, the infective larvae penetrate the skin and enters the body of healthy person.

  From the skin they enter into the blood stream and are carried into the heart and from the heart into the lungs and reach, up to trachea and pharynx from where they are swallowed and reaches to small intestine where they develop into sexually mature worms and starts laying eggs in about six weeks.
- *Symptoms/characteristics/ill effects of hookworm infection*
  i. Iron deficiency anemia
  ii. Joint pains
  iii. Abdominal pains
  iv. Oedema
  v. General weakness
  vi. Loss of body resistance.

- *Preventive and control*
  i. To prevent soil pollution use of sanitary latrines should be promoted in rural areas.
  ii. Defecation in the open area should not be permitted because when the moist soil is contaminated with faeces it leads to development of larvae of hookworm.
  iii. Habit of walking bare-footed should be avoided.
  iv. Sources of water supply should be protected from contamination with human excreta.
  v. Public should be educated for proper use of sanitary latrines as well as personal hygiene especially washing hands after defecation and before taking meals.

Q 14. Describe the cause, mode of transmission, prevention and control of malaria. (S. 96, 99, 00, 02, 03, 04; W. 96, 02, 04, 05, 08)

Malaria

Malaria is a mosquito-born disease cause by the malarial parasite (plasmodium) which belongs to class protozoa.

- *Causative agent*: Malaria is caused by malarial parasites such as:
  i. *Plasmodium vivax*
  ii. *Plasmodium falciparum*
  iii. *Plasmodium malariae*
  iv. *Plasmodium ovale.*
- *Mode of transmission*
  i. Malaria is transmitted by the bite of an infected female anopheles mosquito. During her lifetime a single mosquito may infect several persons. This type of transmission by mosquito is known as vector transmission.
  ii. Malarial parasite may also be transmitted through infected needles and syringes and by blood transfusion.
- *Prevention and control*
  i. Early detection and notification to health authorities.
  ii. Use of drugs such as chloroquine or quinine
  iii. Eliminate mosquito breeding places around houses.
  iv. Do not store water in open container
  v. All water container, coolers, flower pots should be cleaned and dried and then used again.

vi. All drains should be regularly cleaned and sprayed with DDT and BHC.
vii. Kerosene oil should be sprayed over stagnant water so as to kill mosquito larvae.
viii. Larvicidal fish "gambusia fish" should be grown in ponds which will eat mosquito larvae.
ix. Mosquito net, repellants should be used.
x. Health education should be given to the public.

Q 15. Describe the cause, mode of transmission, prevention and control of plague. (S. 97, 98, 02, 03, 06; W. 96, 97, 98, 02, 07)

Plague

Plague is a zoonotic disease, i.e. transmitted from vertebrate animals to men under natural conditions.

- *Causative agent*: The causative agent of plague is *Yersinia pseudotuberculosis, pestis*.
- *Vector*: The vector of plague is rat flea.
- *Mode of transmission*
  i. The *Y. pestis* is transmitted between rodents by fleas. After the death of rat an infected flea may leave the rate and bite a man.
  ii. By direct contact with the tissues of an infected animal.
  iii. By droplet infection, from person to person.
- *Prevention and control*
  i. Early diagnosis and notification to health authorities.
  ii. Isolate the patient and attendants should wear face mask.
  iii. Ensure domestic and personal hygiene.
  iv. Mass destruction of rodents.
  v. Destruction of rat fleas by insecticidal spray.
  vi. Disinfection of sputum, discharge and articles soiled by the patients.
  vii. Immunization with plague vaccine.
  viii. Use of drugs like tetracycline.
  ix. Garbage must be disposed of.
  x. Health education to the public with the facts about plague.
  xi. Dead bodies of plague hit persons should be handled with care.

Q 16. Describe the cause, mode of transmission, prevention and control of filariasis. (S. 08; W. 96, 02, 03)

Filariasis/Lymphatic filariasis

This term is used for infection with three worms (nematodes) namely, *W. bancrofti, B. malayi* and *B. timori*.

- *Causative agent*: Lymphatic filariasis is a mosquito borne disease caused by the filarial parasites *W. bancrofti* and *B. malayi*.
- *Incubation period*: 9 months
- *Mode of transmission*: This infection is transmitted to man by the bite of infected mosquitoes harbouring infective larvae. Two types of mosquitoes transmit the infection:
  - i. Banocroft's filariasis
  - ii. Malayan filariasis.
- *Prevention and control*
  - i. Protection from mosquito bite by using mosquito nets, repellant creams, etc.
  - ii. Early detection and prompt treatment.
  - iii. Use of insecticides, sanitary disposal of wastes, prevention of mosquito breeding.
  - iv. Periodic blood examination.
  - v. Providing hearth education to the public.
  - vi. Diethyl carbamazine (DEC) is the drug of choice for treating filariasis.

Q 17. Describe the cause, mode of transmission, prevention and control of AIDS. (S. 02, 04, 05, 06; W. 96, 97, 98, 99, 02, 05, 06, 07)

AIDS

AIDS is an acquired immunodeficiency syndrome.

- *Causative agent*: AIDs is caused by a virus known as human immunodeficiency virus (HIV).
- *Mode of transmission*
  - i. By sexual contact.
  - ii. Transmission through blood, transfusion, using infected injection, equipment razors, etc.
  - iii. From infected mothers to foetus through, placenta.
  - iv. Through contaminated needles and syringes.
- *Prevention and control*
  - i. Avoiding sex with multiple partners.

ii. Use of condoms during intercourse.
iii. Use of sterilized needles, syringes and surgical equipment.
iv. Screening of blood donors.
v. Blood and blood products should be screened for AIDS before transfusion.
vi. Use of new razors for every person in hair cutting saloons.
vii. Health education to the public regarding dangerous effects of AIDS.

Q 18. Describe the cause, mode of transmission, prevention and control of syphilis. (S. 04; W. 96, 02, 04, 06)

Syphilis

- *Causative agent*: Syphilis is a chronic sexually transmitted infection caused by *Treponema pallidum*.
- *Incubation period*: 9 months.
- *Mode of transmission*
  i. By direct sexual contact.
  ii. Through the placenta infected mothers to its foetus.
  iii. Through infected towels, kissing, etc.
- *Prevention and control*
  i. Avoid sex with multiple partners and prostitutes.
  ii. Detection of positive cases and their thorough treatments.
  iii. Use of condoms to avoid further spread and prevention.
  iv. Health education to public about STD and its problems.

Q 19. Describe the cause, mode of transmission, prevention and control of gonorrhoea. (S. 08; W. 08)

Gonorrhoea

- *Causative agent*: Gonorrhoea is a sexually transmitted disease caused by gram-negative bacteria *Neisseria gonorrhoeae*.
- *Mode of transmission*
  i. By direct sexual contact.
  ii. Through blood transfusion, infected needles and syringes.
  iii. To certain it may spread indirectly through infected towels, bed sheets, clothes, etc. but it is rare since the germs die readily outside the body.
- *Prevention and control*
  i. By avoiding sex with multiple partners and prostitutes.
  ii. Use of condoms during intercourse.

iii. If a positive case is detected, it should be treated thoroughly.
iv. Health education to public about STD and its problems.

Q 20. Describe the cause, mode of transmission, prevention and control of leprosy. (S. 96, 98, 99, 01, 06, 08; W. 02, 03, 04, 08)

Leprosy (Hansens Disease)

- *Causative agent*: Leprosy is chronic communicable disease caused by *Mycobacterium leprae*.
- *Mode of transmission*
  i. Direct contact (body contact) between an infectious patient and a healthy person.
  ii. By indirect contact with fomities such as contaminated clothes and utensils.
  iii. Transmission by droplet infection.
  iv. The bacilli can also be transmitted from breast milk of the infected mother to their infants.
- *Prevention and control*
  i. Early detection and notification of infected cases.
  ii. Isolation of patients in their homes or hospitals.
  iii. The discharges of the pateints, clothes, etc. should be disinfected thoroughly.
  iv. Avoid the contact of children with patient.
  v. Rehabilitation therapy is followed.
  vi. Drugs like dapsone, rifampicin and clofazimine are used.
  vii. Health education to public regarding effects of disease.

Q 21. Describe the cause, mode of transmission, prevention and control of rabies or hydrophobia. (S. 00, 02, 06, 07; W. 96, 98, 07, 08)

Rabies (Hydrophobia)

Rabies is an acute and highly fatal viral infections disease affecting CNS.

Rabies is also known as hydrophobia because the patient show fear from water and is unable to drink water in spite of intense thirst.

Rabies is a disease of warm blooded animals like dogs, cats, monkeys and foxes, etc.

Amongst domestic animals, dog is the commonest source of infection to man.

- *Causative agent*: Rabies is caused by Lyssa virus Type I.
- *Mode of transmission*
  i. Rabies is mainly spread by bites of rabid animals (dog is the common example).
  ii. Saliva of rabid animals is the most common source of infection.
  iii. By leaks on abraded skin or mucosa the virus enters the body. It can travel up the nerves and reaches the rain and causes the disease.
- *Symptoms/clinical features*
  i. Headache, slight fever.
  ii. Pain at the site of wound.
  iii. Saliva runs from mouth.
  iv. Patient cannot tolerate noise and bright light.
  v. Difficulty in swallowing.
  vi. Fear of water.
- *Prevention and control*
  i. Clean the wound and scratches with soap and water as early possible and apply spirit or tract iodine on the wound and cover it with surgical dressing.
  ii. The patient is isolated in a quite dark room.
  iii. Antirabies vaccine is given after exposure.
  iv. The best way to control rabies is to destroy all stray and ownerless dogs and to vaccinate all the pet dogs.

Q 22. Describe the cause, mode of transmission, prevention and control of tetanus. (S. 98, 03, 04, 08; W. 96)

Tetanus

Tetanus is an important acute endemic infection in India.

- *Causative agent*: Tetanus is caused by the endotoxin of *Clostridium tetani*.
- *Mode of transmission*
  i. By contamination of wounds with tetanus spores.
  ii. Injuries caused by iron articles are the major causes of tetanus.
  iii. Tetanus may also occur after injection and vaccinations.
  iv. Tetanus may result from surgery, called as postoperative tetanus.
  v. Other causes includes pin prick, abrasion, wound, burns, human bite, etc.

- *Prevention and control*
  i. Active immunization with tetanus toxoid (TT).
  ii. Infants and children are best immunized by giving DPT vaccine.
  iii. Pregnant women should be given tetanus toxoid doses as a routine to prevent neonatal tetanus.
  iv. Complete sterility precautions should be taken during child birth.
  v. All the wounds should be thoroughly cleaned and long acting penicillins should be administered.

Q 23. Describe the cause, mode of transmission, prevention and control of trachoma. (S.03)

Trachoma

It is a chronic communicable disease of eye and is an important cause of blindness.

- *Causative agent*: Trachoma is caused by a virus called *Chlamydia trachomatis* that attacks mucous membrane covering the surface of the eyeball and lining of eyelids.
- *Mode of transmission*
  i. Direct or indirect contact with ocular discharges of infected persons.
  ii. Contact with infected towels, clothes, handkerchiefs, fingers, etc.
  iii. Swimming pools where water gets contaminated also acts as a source of infection.
  iv. Flies also play a major role in spreading trachoma.
  v. Poor personal hygiene, overcrowding, poverty and malnutrition are the contributory factors to spread this disease.
- *Prevention and control*
  i. Early diagnosis and treatment of the trachoma cases.
  ii. Antifly measures should be taken.
  iii. Common use of eye preparations, towels, handkerchief, etc. should be avoided.
  iv. Maintaining personal hygiene.
  v. Surgical correction to prevent blindness.
  vi. Attempts should be made to remove poverty and malnutrition, overcrowding, etc.
  vii. Health education in order to educate the peoples about use of antibiotics and importance of personal hygiene.

CHAPTER 8

Noncommunicable Diseases

Q 1. Define noncommunicable diseases. Give the causes and prevention and control measures of cancer. (S. 98, 99, 04, 05, 06, 09; W. 96, 97, 98, 99, 01, 03, 04, 06)

Noncommunicable Diseases (S. 95)

The diseases which are not transmitted from man to man, or animal to animal but may be caused due to multiple reasons are called as noncommunicable diseases, e.g. cancer, diabetes, night blindness.

Cancer

Cancer is a group of diseases characterized by abnormal and uncontrolled growth of cells with ability of invade and destroy adjacent tissues and even distant organs.

Causes of Cancer

- Use of tobacco leads to cancer of lung, pharynx, mouth, etc.
- Use of alcohol causes liver cancer, stomach cancer.
- High diet leads to breast cancer.
- Lifestyles, habits, customs also have some relation with cancer.
- Exposure to chemicals like benzene, arsenic, cadmium may cause cancer.
- Sunlight, radiations are related with cancer of skin.
- Air pollution, water pollution also develops cancers.
- Hepatitis B virus can produce cancer of the liver.
- Genetic factors are responsible for developing cancer.
- Use of drugs such as oral contraceptives may produce breast cancer in females.

Prevention/Control of Cancer

Primary Prevention

- Control of tobacco and alcohol consumption.
- Control of air and water pollution.
- Improvement of personal hygiene.
- Reduction in the amount of radiation.
- Protect the workers from industrial carcinogenic chemicals.
- Immunization against hepatitis B virus.
- Testing of food, drugs and cosmetics for their carcinogenic activity.
- Early detection and treatment of precancerous lesions.
- Help of law to control carcinogens.
- Cancer education may help to reduce the chances of cancer.

Secondary Prevention

- Registration of cancer cases in hospitals.
- Early detection by cancer screening.
- Treatment facilities should be available to all cancer patients.

Q 2. Enlist different types of cancer. (S. 06; W. 03)

Types of Cancers

- *Carcinomas*: These are developed from ectodermal or endodermal cells, e.g. skin cancer, brain cancer.
- *Sarcomas*: These cancers develop in connective tissues and mesoderm, e.g. bone cancer.
- *Lymphomas*: These are developed from lymph glands, In this type glands are enlarged lymphocytes are more in numbers.
- *Leukaemias*: It is developed from blood tissue. It is called as blood cancer. WBCs are increased and RBCs are decreased.

Q 3. Give the difference between 'benign tumour' and malignant tumour. (S. 96, 97, 99, 01; W. 01, 05)

Benign tumour	*Malignant tumour*
i. Rate of growth is slow.	i. Rate of growth is fast.
ii. It is a masses of differentiated cells.	ii. It is a masses of undifferentiated cells.
iii. It is enveloped by the fibrous connective tissue sheath.	iii. It is not covered by sheath.

Contd...

Benign tumour	*Malignant tumour*
iv. It is not in contact with neighbouring tissue.	iv. It is in contact with neighbouring tissue.
v. It does not spread in the neighbouring tissues.	v. It spreads in the neighbouring tissues.
vi. Usually not fatal	vi. Fatal unless removed in time.
viii. Examples: Lipoma, L. neurofibroma	vii. Examples: Carcinoma, sarcoma, leukaemias.

Q 4. What is diabetes mellitus? Give the causes and prevention and control of diabetes mellitus. (S. 95, 04, 05, 06, 09; W. 03, 05, 06, 07, 08)

Diabetes Mellitus

Diabetes is a group of diseases characterized by a state of chronic hyperglycemia.

Types of Diabetes Mellitus

- Insulin dependent diabetes mellitus (IDDM) Type 1.
- Noninsulin dependent diabetes mellitus (NIDDM) Type 2.

Causes of Diabetes Mellitus

- Insulin deficiency.
- Excessive in take of alcohol.
- High intake of sugar.
- Viral infection.
- Chemical agents like alloxan which destroy B cells.
- Stress, surgery can also cause disease development.
- Genetic defect.
- Low exercise, rest.
- Renal failure.

Prevention and Control of Diabetes Mellitus

- To avoid consumption of alcohol.
- To take care of obesity.
- To control on diet, e.g. sugar.
- To do maximum exercises.
- To maintain blood glucose level within normal limit.
- To maintain ideal body weight.
- Glucose level should be checked at suitable intervals.

- Be free from stress and strains.
- Marriage counselling to avoid marriages among the persons with family history of diabetes.
- Use of antidiabetic drugs like insulin, phenformin, metformin.

Q 5. What is blindness? Give the causes and prevention and control of blindness. (S. 99, 00, 01, 02, 03, 09; W. 96, 04)

Blindness

A WHO recommended definition of blindness as "blindness is an inability to count fingers at a distance of 3 meters".

Causes of Blindness

- The diseases responsible for causing blindness are:

Cataract	62.6%
Refractive errors	19.7%
Trachoma	NA
Glaucoma	5.8%
Corneal problem	0.9%
Eye tumours	4.7%
Injuries/surgeries	1.2%
Other causes	5.1%

From: Sunderlal et al: *Textbook of Community Medicine*, 2/e. CBS P&D, Delhi, p. 607.

- Peoples working in factories, workshops, welding processes are liable to cause eye injuries.
- Exposure to radiations, X-rays, UV rays can leads to eye injuries.
- Congenital diseases, diabetes, hypertension and diseases of nervous system also produce blindness.
- Severe burns, entry of strong irritants like acids may cause blindness.

Prevention and Control of Blindness

- Improving nutrition, personal hygiene of eye.
- Proper treatment of infectious diseases.
- Persons working in factories, weldings, are provided with vitamin A solution, tetracycline ointment and eye bandages.
- Camps can be organised for cataract operations at villages.
- Eye banks are also available for eye donation.
- Education of the blind in the blind's schools.

- People should be educated regarding diseases of eye and its preventive measures.

Q 6. Classify various cardiovascular agents. (S. 97)

Cardiovascular Diseases (CVS)

These are the diseases related to heart and blood vessels.

Classification

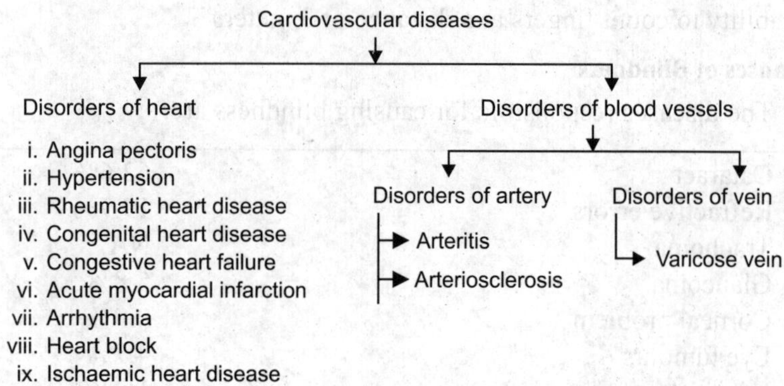

Q 7. Give the causes, prevention and control measures of CVS disorders. (S. 97, 98; W. 96, 00, 01, 02)

Causative/Risk Factors of Cardiovascular Disorders

- Smoking.
- Hypertension.
- High level of serum cholesterol.
- Diabetes.
- Lack of physical activity.
- Alcohol consumption.
- Use of oral contraceptives.
- Age, sex, family history, personality.
- Hereditary.
- Lifestyle, habits.

Preventive Measures, Control and Care of Cardiovascular Disorders

- Reduce fat intake.
- Less consumption of saturated fats.

- Reduction in dietary cholesterol.
- Increase in consumption of vegetables, fruits, etc.
- Avoid alcohol consumption.
- Reduce salt intake.
- Reduce smoking or should be completely restricted.
- Regular physical exercise.
- Control of blood pressure.
- Emotional adjustment, balanced diet, etc.

Q 8. What is hypertension? Give the causes and preventive and control measures of hypertension. (S. 04, 06, 07, 08, 09; W. 98, 03, 05, 06, 07)

Hypertension

The WHO defined hypertension in adult as "a systolic pressure equal to or greater than 160 mmHg and a diastolic pressure equal to or greater than 95 mmHg".

Types of Hypertension

- *Primary hypertension* (*essential hypertension*): It is the type of hypertension of which exact cause is not known. But there is generally a narrowing of blood vessels.
- *Secondary hypertension*: It may be cause due to secondary disorders like renal disorders, endocrine disorders, toxaemia of pregnancy.

Causes of Hypertension (Risk Factors)

- Renal disorders.
- Endocrine disorders.
- Age, genetic factors.
- Obesity, high salt intake.
- Consumption of fatty diet.
- Consumption of alcohol.
- Lack of physical activity.
- Smoking.
- Anxiety or stress.
- Consumption of oral contraceptives.
- Noise and handling of vibrating tools.

Prevention and Control of Hypertension

- Restriction of saturated fat in diet.
- Reduce body weight by promoting exercise.
- Reduce alcohol consumption and smoking.
- Reduce intake of salts.
- Avoid stress, tensions, etc.
- Avoid consumption of excess of oral contraceptives.
- Early detection and treatment.
- Health education and self-care.

CHAPTER 9

Epidemiology

Q 1. Define epidemiology. Give the major uses of epidemiology. (S. 95, 97, 98, 00, 04, 05, 07, 08, 09; W. 96, 97, 98, 02, 03, 08)

Epidemiology

"Epidemiology is the study of distribution and determinants of health related events and diseases in the population and also the application of this knowledge to control health problems."

The term epidemiology is derived from Latin words:
Epi-among, Demons-people, Logos-study.

Uses of Epidemiology/Scope

- It helps to study the disease distribution and its size in the human population.
- It helps for doing community diagnosis and to compare two or more than two geographical areas.
- It helps in planning, implementations and evaluation of health services.
- It helps in the prevention and control of public health problems on priority basis.
- It helps in estimating the needs of resources (money, material, man, etc.)
- It helps in identifying the causes of diseases.
- It helps in identifying clinical syndromes.
- It helps in estimating a person's risk of developing a disease and his chances for survival.

Q 2. Define the terms. (W. 00, 01)

a. Incidence Rate

It is defined as number of new cases of a diseases in a particular geographical area per one thousand population in a defined time period, e.g.

if there are 200 new cases of disease in a population of 40,000 in one year, the incidence rate will be = 200/40,000 ×1000 × 1 = 5 per 1000.

b. Prevalence Rate

It is defined as occurrence of old and new cases of a disease in a particular geographical area per one thousand population in a defined time period, e.g. if 30 new cases of diseases and 40 cases were continuing from last, e.g. if 30 cases of diseases and 40 cases were continuing from last year in the population of 14,000, then prevalence rate will be = (30 + 40)/14,000 × 1000 = 5 per 1000.

Q 3. Define the terms.

- *Infection* (*S. 95, 07*): Infection is defined as the successful entry and development of infectious agent in the host body.
- *Incubation period* (*S. 07; W. 03, 06*): The time interval between entry of disease producing agent into the host body and the appearance of symptoms of disease is called incubation period.
- *Contamination*: It is the presence of infectious agent on inanimate objects such as clothes, beds, toys, utensils, on food items and water.
- *Infestation*: It is defined as lodgement, development and reproduction of arthropod either on body or on the clothing, e.g. lie, mite.
- *Infectious disease*: Any disease resulting from infection is called infectious disease.
- *Contagious disease*: Any disease transmitted by direct or indirect contact is called contagious disease, e.g. scabies, aids.
- *Communicable disease* (*S. 08*): The disease which are transmitted from man to man, animal to animal or man to animal are called communicable diseases, e.g. TB, leprosy.
- *Noncommunicable diseases*: The diseases which are not transmitted from man to man, or animal to animal but may be caused due to multiple reasons are called as noncommunicable diseases, e.g. cancer, diabetes mellitus, night blindness.
- *Epidemic diseases* (*W. 03, 05, 08*): The disease which are rapidly spreading and attacking many peoples in a region in a very short period of time are called epidemic diseases, e.g. smallpox.
- *Endemic disease*: When an infectious disease is always found in certain geographical area, without importation from outside, is termed as endemic disease.

- Sporadic disease (*W. 03, 08*): When a disease occurs at intervals and in single scattered or isolated cases, it is called sporadic disease.
- Pandemic disease: It is the disease present almost in all countries in the world, e.g. AIDS.
- *Zoonotic diseases* (*W. 06, 07*): The diseases which are transmitted from vertebrate animal host to the man under natural conditions are called as zoonotic diseases, e.g. rabies, plague, salmonellosis.
- *Surveillance*: It includes collection, analysis, interpretation and distribution of data related with a disease.
- *Eradication*: It is an absolute term which indicates removal of disease from the complete world.
- *Host* (*W. 08*): A person or animal which allows lodgement of an infectious agent in its body.
- *Fomites*: Fomites are substances capable of absorbing, retaining or transferring infection, e.g. towels, clothes, pens, utensils.
- *Reservoir*: A reservoir is a person or animal or artropod or plant or soil, water and food in which infectious agent is maintained.
- *Carriers*: Carrier are the person who harbour pathogenic micro-organisms of a specific infectious disease without showing any signs and symptoms of the disease but are able to infect other individuals.
- *Source of infection*: The source of infection is defined as "the person, animal or object or substance from which an infectious agent passes to the host".
- *Vector*: A vector is an arthropod or a living animal that transfer the infectious agent to a susceptible individual, e.g. mosquito vector in malaria, filariasis, rat flea in plague.

Q 4. Describe the modes/routes/methods of transmission of communicable diseases/infectious diseases. (S. 96, 97, 98, 02, 04, 07; W. 97, 98, 99, 02, 03, 06)

Modes of transmission of diseases

- A. Air-borne transmission
  - Direct droplet infection
  - Droplet nuclei infection
  - Infected dust
- B. Direct transmission
  - Direct contact
  - Vertical/translatal infection
- C. Indirect transmission
  - Vehicle borne transmission
  - Vector borne transmission
  - Fomite borne transmission

A. Air-borne Transmission

In respiratory infections while patient coughs or sneezes, a shower of small droplets of saliva is generated and dispersed in the atmosphere and there droplets contains thousands of microorganisms and if they are inhaled by a healthy person he gets infected. Droplet infection is possible in three ways:

i. *Direct droplet infection*: In this case, the large droplets may infect the healthy person as they are inhaled directly from the air and because they do not travel long. The mode of transmission requires close contact. Sometimes these droplets fall down on objects like beds, clothing, or dust and may contaminate these articles which may infect the healthy host.

ii. *Droplet nucleic infection*: When the droplets are tiny the moisture content evaporates rapidly and leave behind a minute residue or nucleus which becomes light and remain suspended in the air, which is termed as *droplet nuclei*.

   A droplet nuclei may contain one or many organism. This nucleus remains in the atmosphere and may be transferred to other place by wind and whenever it is inhaled by a healthy host it may infect the host. Droplet nuclei may survive in atmosphere for a considerable period of time.

iii. *Infected dust*: In this case droplets settle down on articles or fall down on the dust. This infected dust is elevated in the air while dry sweeping bed making and may inhaled by the host and can get infected.

B. Direct Transmission

When no external agency is required for the transmission of infection is called as direct transmission.

i. *Direct contact:* Infection is transmitted by direct contact of skin of two persons. The contact may be by touching or by sexual intercourse or living very close to an infected person, e.g. eye infections, leprosy, AIDS.

ii. *Vertical or transplacental infections*: When the disease agent is transmitted from infected mother to the foetus, it is called vertical or transplacental transmission, e.g. AIDS, Hepatitis-B, Rubella virus.

C. Indirect Transmission

If transmission of disease agent requires some substance like milk, water insect or some belonging of the patient it is called indirect transmission. The inanimate substances during the process of transmission are called "vehicle" and the insect is called "vector" of the disease:

i. *Vehicle borne transmission*: The commonest vehicle for disease transmission is water and such diseases, are called "water borne diseases", e.g. cholera, typhoid, diarrhoea, dysentery.

   Other important vehicles are milk, raw fruits, vegetables, blood products, tissues, organs, e.g. milk borne diseases diphtheria, sore throat, enteric fever.

ii. *Vector borne transmission*: A vector is an arthropod or a living animal that transfers the infectious agent to a susceptible host.

   Vector borne transmission is very simple as flies transmit the disease agents from one place to another on their bodies, wings or legs, e.g. mosquito vector takes part in the life cycle of the disease agent for example, in malaria, filariasis, rat flea is a vector of plague.

iii. *Fomite borne transmission*: Fomites are the belonging of the patient which come in direct contact with the patient and get contaminated. Fomites includes clothes, towels, utensils, pens, instruments and removed dressing. These fomites can preserve the disease agent. For sometimes and whenever a healthy person uses these articles, the disease agent is transmitted to him.

Q 5. Define host. What are the types of host?

Host

"Host is a person or animal which allows lodgement of an infectious agent in his body."

Types of Host

- *Obligate host*: It means as man in meascles or typhoid where no animal host exists.
- *Intermediate host*: The host in which asexual part of life cycle of the parasite takes place.
- *Definite host*: The host in which sexual part of life cycle of the parasite takes place.

- *Susceptible host*: It means man which easily allows the microorganisms to establish either on the tissues or within the body to cause infection.

Q 6. What is reservoir? Explain types of reservoir of infection.

Reservoir

"A reservoir is a person or animal or arthropod or plant or soil, water and food in which infectious agent is maintained."

Types of Reservoir

- *Human reservoir*: It can be a case suffering from the particular disease but an infect others. They can be identified by laboratory examinations.

  In some diseases the infective agent remains in the body without the disease because of various reasons as improper treatment, low resistance, immune disorders.
- *Animal reservoir*: The diseases which primarily affect animals but can also infect human beings are called zoonotic disease, e.g. rabies (hydrophobia), influenza, yellow fever. The occurrence of this disease depends upon the migration of animals from one place to another.
- *Nonliving reservoir*: This can be soil, water, food fruits and vegetables, milk products, contaminated objects like furnitures, stationary, clothing, linen, utensils, formites, etc. and laboratory materials including surgical instruments. The disease agent can be virus, bacteria, rickettsiae.

Q 7. Define carriers. What are the types of disease carriers? (S. 07)

Carriers

Carrier is defined as the person or any animal carrying the disease agent but not showing any sign and symptom of disease but are able to infect other individuals.

Types of Disease Carriers

- *Incubation carriers*: These are the persons during incubation period of the infetious disease.
- *Contact carriers*: These are persons who are in contact with a case of an infectious disease and carry microbes morphologically identical with those causative of the diseases.

- *Convalescent carriers*: These are persons who continue to harbour during convalescence. They are sometimes called acute carriers.
- *Chronic carriers*: These are persons who harbour infective organisms for a long period (e.g. 3 months) after recovery from the disease. Such carriers are more dangerous.

Q 8. What are "hospital acquired infections"? How are they prevented?/ Nosocomial infections. (S. 95, 98, 00, 01, 04, 07, 08; W. 01, 03, 06, 07)

Nosocomial Infections

"It is an infection appearing in a patient when he or she visited the hospital or other health care facility."

It is not related with disease for with patient was admitted. In other words, if the patient had not visited the hospital, the patient would have no acquired the infection. The symptoms may appear after his discharge from the hospital. It is reported that about 5% of patients admitted to the hospitals are likely to get such infections.

Sources/Causes of Nosocomial Infection

- Staff attending the patient such as sweepers, nurses, doctors suffering from infection.
- Cross infection from other person in hospital who are already infected.
- Persons visiting the hospitals to see the patients.
- Due to objects like surgical instruments, dressing, etc.
- Due to infected syringe and needles.

Examples of Hospital Acquired Infections

- Hepatitis-B
- HIV infection
- UT infections
- Wound infections
- Tuberculosis
- Pneumonia.

Prevention and Control of "Hospital Acquired Infections"

- Patients with infections should be isolated.
- Disinfecting the air in hospital.
- Avoid spitting and smoking in hospital.
- The surrounding environment of the patient should be kept completely from dust which may spread infection.

- Articles used by patients should be disinfected.
- Aseptic measures should be followed in wards, operation theatres, labour rooms.
- All the cases of wound infection should be notified.
- There should be adequate space between beds.
- Cleaning and sterilization of urine pots, kidney-trays bed-pans should be done regularly.
- UV lamps should be provided.
- All the staff attending patients, should have periodical medical check to detect and treat infection.
- Every hospital should have an infection control committee which should monitor and control infections in a hospital.

Q 9. What do you mean by notifiable diseases? Give examples.

Notifiable Diseases

The diseases which should be immediately intimated to the local health authorities to take preventive measures and to provide medical care to the patients, are called as notifiable diseases.

Example

- Cholera
- Smallpox
- Plague
- Leprosy
- Tuberculosis
- Whooping cough
- Meascles
- Typhoid, etc.

Q 10. What do you mean by notification of diseases? Give its advantages/uses/importance/significance.

Notification

Notification is a procedure required to report the occurrence of every notifiable disease to the health authority at earliest.

- Notification is one of the preventive measures taken up to control spread of disease.
- Notification indicates immediate intimation of every case of an infectious disease to the available healthy authority such as

municipal medical officer of health, district medical officer of health.

Advantages/Importance of Notification

- It allows the authorities to isolate the patient, to treat patient and to follow necessary disinfection.
- It helps to prevent the spread of infection by promptly taking measures and thus safeguard the rest of the community by vaccination.
- The real and original source of infection can be found out and corrected.
- It helps to control spread of infection through schools or other centre by excluding members of infected household.
- It provides, an opportunity of investigation of the sanitary condition of all households, where diseases are reported.
- It provides opportunity of investigation the source of an epidemic by examining milk supplies, water supplies, etc.

Q 11. What is the isolation of patient? How isolation of patient is done in hospital and private houses?

Isolation of Patient

"It means complete separation of infected person from contact of other human beings for the period of communicability."

- Isolation can be done either in hospitals or at homes.
- The period of isolation depends upon the degree of spreading ability of infected person.
- The purpose of isolation is to protect the community from infectious disease.

A. *Isolation Hospital*

1. The site of hospital should be dry, healthy, and well-drained.
2. It should be away from congested area.
3. It should have convenient approach.
4. Separate wards should be provided for different infectious diseases.
5. Each patient should have 144 square feets floor space and 6000 cubic feet of fresh air per hour.
6. There should be proper arrangement for the supply of pure water, removal of excreta and urine.
7. Soiled clothes should properly disinfected.

B. *House Isolation/Home Isolation*

- The sick room should be separated and should be located at upper floor.
- All necessary furniture should be removed.
- A sheet soaked in a disinfectant should be hung in front of the door as a curtain.
- The windows should be kept open to ensure adequate ventilation.
- Only attendants or nurses should be allowed to go in the sick room. They must wash their hands in some disinfectant solution before leaving the sick room.
- The soiled clothes of the patient should be immersed in disinfectant solution and then boiled.
- Excreta and remainder of food should be received in a vessel containing a strong disinfectant solution and should be buried in the ground or burnt away.
- Anti-fly and anti-mosquito measures must be taken to exclude flies and mosquitoes from the sickroom.
- The utensils must be disinfected properly after taking them out of the sick room.
- Visitors should not be allowed to enter the sickroom.
- Children and workers from the infected house should not be allowed to go to their respective institutions.
- After being out of danger of infection, the patient should be well washed and bathed thoroughly and given a complete charge of clothes before mixing with other persons.
- In case of death, the dead body should be recovered in a sheet soaked in carbolic solution and burned as soon as possible.
- The sick room should be thoroughly disinfected after having been vacated by the patient.

Q 12. Define the terms.

- *Antiseptic*: Any substance which destroy or inhibits the growth of microbes which applied to living tissue is called antiseptic.
- *Disinfectant*: Any substance which destroy or microbes but not usually spores when applied to nonliving objects.
- *Sterilisation*: It is the process of complete destruction of micro-organisms from the system.
- *Disinfection*: It is the process of destruction of disease causing agent from the inanimate objects.

Q 13. Explain the recommended "disinfection procedures" for the following.

a. Faeces and Urine (Stools) (S. 98, 02, 03, 07; W. 01, 02, 07)

- Faeces and urine should be collected in impervious containers.
- Equal volume of –10% bleaching powder solution is added.
- Phenol, cresol (5%), formalin (10%) may be used.
- It is kept for 2 hours.
- Alternatively quick lime solution 20–25% can be used as a substitute.
- Some times only boiling water can be used for disinfection.
- The containers of urine and stools are disinfected with 2–3% cresol solution.
- If possible containers are disinfected by steam.

b. Sputum (S. 98, 99, 00, 04, 06; W. 02, 03, 07)

- Sputum is collected in paper containers.
- It is disinfected by burning on small scale.
- If the amount is large (as in TB hospitals) then it is boiled under pressure (20 pounds) for ½ an hour and then buried.
- Readymade papercups containing cresol solution may be given to the patient.
- The patient may spit in that cup containing cresol solution and the cup is kept for 2 hours and then disposed of.

c. Rooms (S. 95, 97; W. 03)

- When rooms are properly, cleaned and well ventilated by exposure to direct sunlight, are naturally disinfected.
- Cresol (2%) formaldehyde (1%), concentration solution of bleaching powder are used to disinfect the rooms.
- The floor and walls are mopped with the soaps and water solution and then room is washed after 4 to 6 hours.
- For operation theatres the air inside the room should be disinfected and formalin fumes are used.
- Potassium permanganate powder is added to formalin solution and in the mixture of 1 litre, water is added. Then it is boiled and fumes generated are allowed to spread into the closed room. The room is kept closed for 12 hours and then it can be used.
- Alternatively 500 ml of formalin mixed with 1 litre of water is boiled and the fumes are generated.

d. Linen and Beddings (S. 97, 06, 08)

- Bed sheets and other linen articles soiled with infected materials are washed with soap and water.
- These are treated with a disinfectant (cresol 2–3%) and then are boiled for 20–30 minutes in water and soap is added for better action.
- Bed sheets and linen articles are also autoclaved after washing or ionising radiations are used.
- Sometimes bed sheets and linen articles are washed in hot water and put in sun to prevent cross-infection.

e. Instruments (S. 97)

- Boiling in lane water or autoclaving is the most suitable method for disinfection of surgical instruments like scissors, scalpel and blunt instruments.
- Syringes and glass articles which are not used for surgical operations can be disinfected by boiling for about 30 minutes.
- Boiling cannot kill the spores, so chemical disinfection with either cresols solution is also practiced.
- Instruments used for surgery are autoclaved.
- Plastic instruments are disinfected by chemicals.
- Very sharp and sophisticated instruments are sterilized in hot air oven or by ionising radiations.

f. Dead Bodies (S. 03, 04)

- Dead bodies should be wrapped in a powerful disinfectant.
- Burying: The dead bodies are buried under the earth in a marked area called graveyard situated at the periphery of city or town.
- Burning: It is done by wood or by an electric furnace.

Q 14. Define disinfection. Describe the types of disinfection. (S. 99, 01, W. 96, 05, 06)

Disinfection

Disinfection is the process of destruction of disease causing agent from an inanimate object.

Types of Disinfection

- *Concurrent disinfection*: It means immediate application of disinfective measures after the discharge of infectious material from the body of an infected person.

Concurrent disinfection is more commonly practised in hospitals. Spoiled clothes, linen bed sheets, dressing, aprons and gloves are treated with the disinfectant as soon as they are spoiled.

- *Terminal disinfection*: It is the application of disinfective measures after the patient has been removed by death or to a hospital.
  This involves the disinfection of bed, furniture, bed sheets and rooms of the patient.
- *Precurrent* (*prophylactic*) *disinfection*: Disinfection of water by chlorine, pasteurization of milk, handwashings are the examples of precurrent disinfection.
- *Natural disinfection*: Sunlight is a very good disinfectant for many things like rooms furniture, linen, etc.

Natural disinfection mesures are useful but are not sufficeint.

Q 15. Discuss different methods of disinfection. (W. 00, 04)

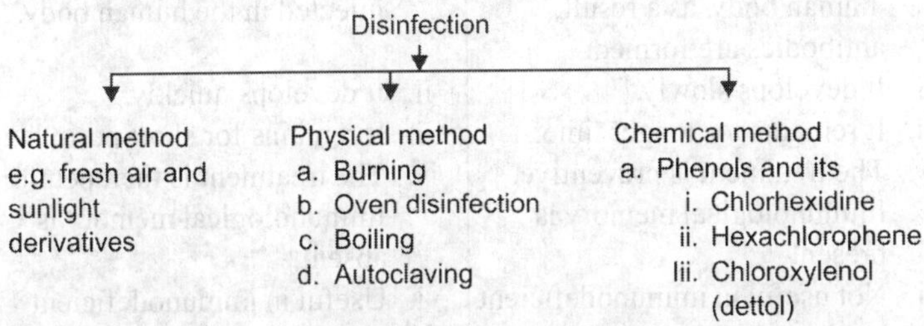

Q 16. Define and classify immunity. Enlist various immunising agents. (S. 96, 97, 99, 00, 01, 09; W. 98, 01)

Immunity

Immunity is the power of the body to resist the effect of invasion of pathogenic microorganisms in the body.

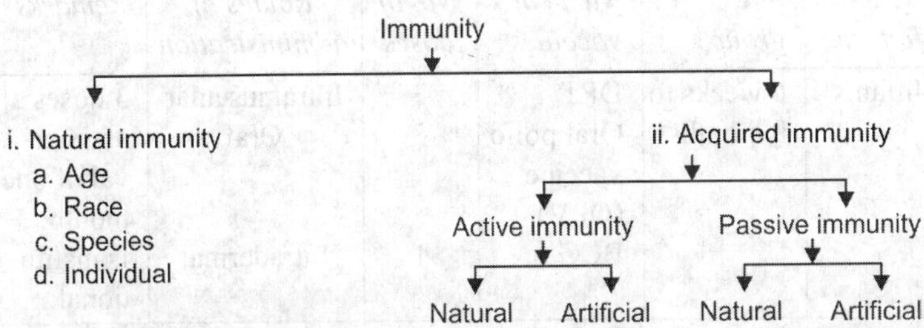

Immunising Agents

- Vaccines
  - i. Live vaccines
  - ii. Inactivated (killed) vaccines
  - iii. Toxoids
  - iv. Cellular fractions
  - v. Combined vaccines.
- Immunoglobulins
  - i. Normal human immunoglobulins
  - ii. Special human immunoglobulins.
- Antisera or antitoxins.

Q 17. Give the difference between active and passive immunity. (S. 05; W. 97, 98, 03, 07)

Active immunity	*Passive immunity*
i. Antigens are injected in the human body, as a result, antibodies are formed.	i. Readymade antibodies are injected in the human body.
ii. It develops slowly.	ii. It develops quickly.
iii. It remains for longer time.	iii. It remains for short period.
iv. The treatment is preventive.	iv. The treatment is therapeutic.
v. Immunological memory is present.	v. Immunological memory is absent.
vi. Not useful in immunodeficient hosts.	vi. Useful in immunodeficient host.
vii. No inheritance	vii. May be acquired from mother.
viii. Preparations, e.g. vaccine, toxoids.	viii. Preparation: Sera.

Q 18. State the national immunisation schedule. (S. 04, 07, 09; W. 04, 05)

Beneficiaries	*Age group*	*Name of vaccines*	*No. of doses*	*Routes of administration*	*Remarks*
Infants	6 weeks to 9 months	DPT Oral polio vaccine (OPV) BCG	3 3 1	Intramuscular Oral Intradermal	3 doses at an interval of one month. Is institutional

Contd...

Beneficiaries	*Age group*	*Name of vaccines*	*No. of doses*	*Routes of administration*	*Remarks*
					delivery BCG can be given at birth.
	9–12 months	Measles	1	Subcutaneous	
Children	16–24 months	DPT (I Boaster)	1	Intramuscular	
		OPV (I Booster)	1	Oral	
	5–6 years	DT (II Booster)	1	Intramuscular	2 dose if not immunized previously
		Typhoid	2	Subcutaneous	At an interval of one month.
10 years		Tetanus toxoid (TT)	1	Intramuscular	2 doses if not immunized previously.
16 years		Tetanus toxoid (TT)	1	Intramuscular	2 dose if not immunized previously
		Typhoid	1	Subcutaneous	2 doses if not immunized previously.
Pregnant women	16–36 weeks	Tetanus toxoid	2	Intramuscular	Only one dose needed if immunized previously within last three years.

Q 19. Give the long forms of following:

HIV	Human Immunodeficiency Virus
AIDS	Acquired Immunodeficiency Syndrome
STD	Sexually Transmitted Diseases
BCG	Bacillus Calmette-Guérin
DPT	Toxoid of Diphtheria and Tetanus
DT	Diphtheria and Toxin
MMR	Measles, Mumps and Rubeola combined vaccine
TAB	Typhoid and Paratyphoid A and B
OPV	Oral Polio Vaccine
TT	Tetanus Toxoid
UTI	Urinary Tract Infection
RTI	Respiratory Tract Infection
GIT	Gastrointestinal Tract
CHD	Congestive Heart Failure
IUD	Intrauterine Device
WHO	World Health Organization
ORS	Oral Rehydration Salt

Q 20. Name the diseases transmitted by following:

- **Air born diseases (S. 04, 09; W. 08)**
  - i. Tuberculosis
  - ii. Measles
  - iii. Chickenpox
  - iv. Whooping cough
  - v. Influenza
  - vi. Diphtheria.
- **Water born diseases (S. 04, 08, 09; W. 04, 08)**
  - i. Cholera
  - ii. Dysentery
  - iii. Typhoid
  - iv. Amoebiasis
  - v. Viral hepatitis
  - vi. Poliomyelitis
  - vii. Viral hepatitis
  - viii. Hookworm infestation.
- **Fomite born diseases**
  - i. Tuberculosis
  - ii. Leprosy

iii. Cholera
iv. Typhoid
v. Plague
vi. Influenza
vii. Whooping cough
viii. Measles.

- **Soil born diseases**
  i. Diarrhoea
  ii. Amoebiasis
  iii. Cholera
  iv. Dysentery
  v. Hookworm diseases.
- **Zoonotic diseases (S. 08)**
  i. Rabies
  ii. Anthrax
  iii. Plague
  iv. TB
  v. Brucellosis.
- **Diseases transmitted by rodents (S. 08)**
  i. Plague
  ii. Ringworm
  iii. Rat bite fever
  iv. Lassa fever
  v. Amoebiasis
  vi. Salmonellosis.
- **Diseases spread by arthropods (S. 04, 08, 09)**
  i. Malaria
  ii. Plague
  iii. Typhoid
  iv. Filariasis.
- **Diseases spread by animals**
  i. Plague
  ii. Tuberculosis
  iii. Leprosy
  iv. Hookworm infestations.
- **Diseases caused by viruses**
  i. Hepatitis
  ii. AIDS

iii. Poliomyelitis
iv. Chickenpox
v. Smallpox
vi. Rabies
vii. Influenza
viii. Measles

- **Diseases caused by bacteria**
  i. Tuberculosis
  ii. Leprosy
  iii. Cholera
  iv. Typhoid
  v. Plague.
- **Diseases caused by fungi**
  i. Candidiasis
  ii. Dermatophytes
  iii. Onychomycosis.
- **Diseases caused by protozoa**
  i. Malaria
  ii. Amoebiasis
  iii. Diarrhoea
  iv. Vaginitis
  v. Uretenitis
  vi. Dysentery.
- **Diseases carried by sand fly**
  i. Kalaazar
  ii. Sand fly fever
  iii. Onychomycosis.
- **Diseases carried by house fly**
  i. Diarrhoea
  ii. Dysentery
  iii. Typhoid
  iv. Paratyphoid
  v. Cholera
  vi. Amoebiasis.
- **Diseases carried by mosquitoes**
  i. Malaria
  ii. Filaria
  iii. Yellow fever.

- **Sexually transmitted diseases (S. 04)**
  1. AIDS
  2. Syphilis
  3. Gonorrhoea.
- **Noncommunicable diseases (S. 04)**
  1. Cancer
  2. Blindness
  3. Diabetes.
- **Surface infections (S. 04, 09)**
  1. Rabies
  2. Trachoma
  3. Tetanus
  4. Leprosy.

Board Question Papers

(From Summer 1997 to Summer 2017)

Summer Examination 1997

D Pharm First Year

Health Education and Community Pharmacy

Q 1. Answer any *five* of the following:

a. State two infectious diseases each carried by insects:
   i. Mosquitoes   ii. House fly

b. State the composition of pure air with their importance.

c. When the water is said to be polluted?

d. Give the important sources of carbohydrates and proteins.

e. Name the disease caused due to deficiency of vitamin A and vitamin B_2.

f. What does the following abbreviations stand for:
   i. BCG   iii. STD
   ii. DPT   iv. AIDS

g. Match the following:

A	B
Vitamins	Deficiency disease caused
i. Calciferol	1. Beriberi
ii. Nicotinic acid	2. Scurvy
iii. Thiamine	3. Rickets
iv. Ascorbic acid	4. Pellagra

Q 2. Answer any *four* of the following:

a. What is disease? Discuss in short the various concepts of prevention of diseases.

b. What are amino acids? Name of the essential amino acids.
c. What programmes related to family planning have been developed by government of India?
d. Define the term health. State and explain in short the aspects of health.
e. What is family planning? What are the objectives of family planning?
f. Describe the important structural features of bacteria with the help of well labelled diagram.

Q 3. Answer any *four* of the following:

a. Define the term first aid. State the scope and major principles of first aid.
b. What are burns and scalds? Give the details of first aid in Burns and Scalds.
c. Name the glands and their hormones which play important role in reproduction.
d. Elaborate the biological treatment of sewage.
e. What are the differences between infectious hepatitis and serum hepatitis?
f. Define the term microbiology. State the different methods for isolation of bacteria.

Q 4. Answer any *five* of the following:

a. Give the source of infection, prevention and control of tuberculosis.
b. Classify different types of cardiovascular diseases along with their cause, prevention and control.
c. Why the bacteria are stained? Explain the method of gram staining.
d. Define demography. State the different stages of population growth cycle.
e. Define food poisoning. State its different types prevention and control in general.
f. What is shock? Describe the first aid treatment in shock.

Q 5. Answer any *five* of the following:

a. What do you mean by determinants of health? State various factors which determines the health?
b. What is a balanced diet? What are the common deficiency in Indian diet?
c. What are the different methods of contraception? Classify them with examples.
d. What are different types of fracture? Describe the general first aid treatment for fractures.

e. Describe any two major types of fungal diseases.
f. Discuss the modes of transmission of infectious diseases.

Q 6. Answer any *four* of the following:

a. What is benign tumour and malignant tumour? State classification of caner.
b. Give the causative agent, mode of transmission, prevention and control of plague.
c. Define the term epidemiology. What are the uses of epidemiology?
d. Discuss the disinfection procedures for:
   i. Linen
   ii. Room
   iii. Instruments
e. Define the term immunity. Discuss the classification with examples.
f. What is virus? Elaborate major types of viruses and diseases caused by them.

Winter Examination 1997

D Pharm First Year

Health Education and Community Pharmacy

Q 1. Answer the following questions:

a. Name the causative agent of the following diseases (any *two*):
   i. Diphtheria
   ii. Gonorrhoea
   iii. Malaria
b. Name the disease caused due to deficiency of the following (any *two*):
   i. Vitamin B
   ii. Iodine
   iii. Fats
c. Answer any *two*:
   i. Name one disease spread by rodents.
   ii. Name one disease spread by animals.
   iii. Name one disease spread by arthopods.
d. Answer any *two*:
   i. Name one airborne disease.
   ii. Name one disease spread by arthropods.
   iii. Name one fomite borne disease.

e. Define any *two*:
   i. Health education
   ii. Community pharmacy
   iii. Microbiology.

Q 2. Answer any *four* of the following:

a. Define health. What are the signs of a helathy person?
b. Explain the role of carbohydrates in our food.
c. What is demography? Explain demographic cycle.
d. What first should be given to a burn case?
e. What is safe water? Enumerate the different sources of water.
f. Give a short classification of microbes.

Q 3. Answer any *four* of the following:

a. What is the mode of transmission of whooping cough? How can it be prevented?
b. What is cancer? How can it be controlled?
c. What is epidemiology? What are the major types of epidemics?
d. What is primary prevention? Explain with example. What are its advantages?
e. What are the qualities of an ideal contraceptive?
f. How will you handle a patient who has swallowed poison?

Q 4. Answer any *four* of the following:

a. What is "solid waste"? Give a short account of the methods of waste disposal.
b. What is meant by "culture media"; "pure culture technique" and "streak and spread plate technique"?
c. What are the different types of food poisoning? How can it be controlled?
d. What is diabetes? What are its preventive measures?
e. Explain the difference between active immunity and passive immunity.
f. What is malnutrition? What are its causes?

Q 5. Answer any *four* of the following:

a. What are barrier methods of family planning? State its advantages and disadvantages.
b. What is an open fracture? How will you handle a person with a fracture in the arm?
c. Compare composting and trenching.
d. Explain "pathogenic bacteria". Give two examples with their staining techniques.

e. What is the causative agent of typhoid? Describe the mode of transmission of the disease.
f. What are the general principles of disease prevention?

Q 6. Answer any *four* of the following:

a. What is the role of folic acid in the body? Explain.
b. Explain the mode of transmission plague? Name the drugs used to combat plague.
c. What is meant by 'AIDS'? What are its mode of transmission and control?
d. Give a short account of dynamics of disease transmission.
e. What do you mean by family planning? Mention the advantages and disadvantages of hormonal contraceptives.
f. What is medical entomology? What are the principles of arthropod control?

Summer Examination 1998

D Pharm First Year

Health Education and Community Pharmacy

Q 1. Answer any *five* of the following:

a. State the main sources of water supply.
b. Give the advantages and disadvantages of condom.
c. Give the composition of pure air with its importance.
d. Give the uses of amino acids. Discuss its types.
e. State the causative agent and symptoms of measles.
f. What are helath determinants, explain suitably?
g. Match the following:

A	B
Minerals	Deficiency diseases
i. Iron	1. Hypothyroidism
ii. Zinc	2. Anaemia
iii. Iodine	3. Dental caries
iv. Flourine	4. Growth retardation
	5. Skin disorders

Q 2. Answer any *four* of the following:

a. Define the term epidemiology. What is the importance of epidemiology?
b. What are the different forms of plague? Give the organism, mode of transmission and methods to control plague.

c. What are the sign and symptoms of heart-attacks? Describe the first aid treatment in heart-attack.
d. What is family welfare? What are the objectives of family welfare programme?
e. Define the term microbiology? State any two types of classification of microorganism.
f. What is balanced diet? What are the deficiencies in Indian diet?

Q 3. Answer any *four* of the following:

a. What is virus? Name two diseases caused by viruses.
b. Discuss the common modes of transmission of an infectious.
c. Define the term first aid. State the aim and major principles of first aid.
d. State the different types of hepatitis with causative agents. Give the mode of transmission and control of hepatitis A and B.
e. State the different types of STD. Discuss the pathological features and control measures of syphilis.
f. What are the ill-effects of sunlight? State the various method to control them.

Q 4. Answer any *four* of the following:

a. Explain in short the various factors that increase the susceptibility of the person to cancer.
b. What are air-borne infections? Elaborate causes of hospital acquired infections.
c. Discuss the methods for small scale purification of water. What are the disadvantages of hard water?
d. Describe coitus interruptus method of family planning with its advantages and disadvantages.
e. What are communicable diseases? Write the causative organism, mode of transmission and symptoms of leprosy.
f. Describe method of preventing modes of transmission and causative organism of tuberculosis.

Q 5. Answer any *four* of the following:

a. Enlist the types of fat soluble vitamins. State the sources and functions of vitamin A.
b. Describe the first aid treatment for snakebite.
c. Name three major types of arthropod borne diseases.
d. Write a short note on mouth-to-mouth respiration.
e. State the major types of fungal diseases. Discuss candidiasis.
f. What is tetanus? State in short the different methods of prevention of tetanus.

Q 6. Answer any *four* of the following:

a. Define the term disinfection. Discuss the disinfection procedures for:

   i. Sputum   ii. Faeces

b. What are proteins? Give their sources and functions.

c. Write a note on kwashiorkor disease.

d. Define the term health. Name the various indicators of health.

e. Write a short note on acid-fast staining.

f. What are the causative agents and methods of prevention of diabetes?

Winter Examination 1998

D Pharm First Year

Health Education and Community Pharmacy

Q 1. Answer any *five* of the following:

a. Define the term mortality and morbidity.

b. Give the sources and deficiency diseases of iron and calcium.

c. What are the natural methods for temporary contraception?

d. State the two diseases each carried by sand flies and house flies.

e. Give the composition of air. State its importance.

f. Fill in the blank suitably any two:

   i. Influenza is caused by the virus ________.

   ii. The deficiency of iodine causes ________.

   iii. Habitual occurrence of a disease within a given geographic area is known as ________.

   iv. The treatment of diseases with the anti-infective drug is known as ________.

g. Match the following:

A	B
Vitamin D	Thiamine
Vitamin E	Calciferol
Vitamin B_1	Ascorbic acid
Vitamin C	Tocopherols

Q 2. Answer any *four* of the following:

a. List out the major sources of water pollution. How the pollution of water can be prevented or controlled?

b. What is hydrophobia? State the symptoms and give the methods of prevention and control of rabies.

c. Define microbiology? What are the different methods for isolation of bacteria?
d. What is cancer? State the measures for prevention and control of cancer.
e. What is hypertension? What are the causes of hypertension?
f. Define the term immunity. Differentiate between active and passive immunity?

Q 3. Answer any *four* of the following:

a. Write a short note on burns and scalds.
b. State the procedure employed in minor surgery and dressing.
c. Write a note on acid-fast staining.
d. State the different types of hepatitis with causative agent. Give the symptoms, mode of transmission and control of hepatitis-A.
e. Discuss the disinfection procedures for:
   i. Room
   ii. Linen
   iii. Instruments
f. Discuss the modes of transmission of infectious agent.

Q 4. Answer any *four* of the following:

a. Define epidemiology. What is the importance of epidemiology?
b. Describe the first aid treatment for snakebite.
c. What are splints? What are the different types of splints?
d. Write a note on sound-pollution.
e. What is food poisoning? Discuss the general preventive measures and treatment for poisoning.
f. Give the causative organism, symptoms, mode of transmission and control for tuberculosis.

Q 5. Answer any *four* of the following:

a. How the biological treatment of sewage is done?
b. What are the different types of veneral diseases? State the diagnostic characters and mode of transmission of AIDS.
c. What are fats? Give the sources and functions of fats.
d. Write a short note on Wilson's disease.
e. What is disease? Discuss in short the various concepts of prevention of diseases.
f. How the pharmacist can promote the family planning?

Q 6. Answer any *four* of the following:

a. Discuss the various indicators that are used for the assessment of health.
b. Write a short note on hormonal contraceptives.

c. Give the organism (causative), mode of transmission, prevention and control for plague.
d. Define the term first-aid. State the principles and discuss the scope of first aid.
e. State the major types of fungal diseases. Discuss any two of them.
f. Differentiate between communicable and noncommunicable diseases.

Summer Examination 1999

D Pharm First Year

Health Education and Community Pharmacy

Q 1. Answer any *five* of the following:

a. Define mental health and social health.
b. What are vitamins and minerals.
c. Define the term immunity. State its types.
d. State the disinfection procedure for infected sputum.
e. State the disadvantages of hard water.
f. State the factors affecting fertility.
g. State the ill effects of noise.

Q 2. Answer any *four* of the following:

a. What are proteins? Name the essential amino acids.
b. What is ventilation? State the various types of ventilation. Give the uses of ventilation.
c. Explain the concept of prevention of diseases.
d. State the different forms of beriberi. Discuss dry beriberi.
e. What is family planning? Define its goals.
f. What are different types of fractures? Describe the general first aid treatment for fractures.

Q 3. Answer any *four* of the following:

a. Classify the sources of water. Name the various water-borne diseases.
b. Describe general structural features of virus with the help of a labelled diagram.
c. Give the causative agent, mode of transmission, prevention and control of typhoid.
d. What is balanced diet? State the common faults in Indian diet.
e. Name various methods of family planning with suitable examples.
f. Describe the first aid treatment in case of snakebite.

Q 4. Answer any *four* of the following:

a. Write a note on rapid-sand filter.
b. Describe in brief the various methods of disposal of solid waste.
c. Explain the cause of night-blindness. Discuss its prevention and treatment.
d. Give the causative agent, mode of transmission, prevention and control of syphilis.
e. What are arthropod-borne diseases? Describe the causes and control of malaria.
f. State the various techniques of staining bacteria. Give the method of acid-fast staining.

Q 5. Answer any *four* of the following:

a. Name the glands, their hormones and functions which play important role in reproduction.
b. Write a note on immunoglobulins.
c. What is sewage? What are the aims of sewage treatment.
d. Define the term microbiology. State the methods for isolation of bacteria.
e. Give the causative agent, characteristic features and forms of leprosy. State the deformities produced by leprosy.
f. What is benign tumour and malignant tumour? State the various causes for cancer.

Q 6. Answer any *four* of the following:

a. What are respiratory infections? Name the various types of respiratory infections.
b. What is disinfection? Discuss in brief different types of disinfection methods.
c. Write a note on role of pharmacist in family planning.
d. Name the various rodents and the diseases transmitted by them. How rodent borne diseases are transmitted?
e. Discuss the design and mechanism of septic tank.
f. Write a note on resuscitation.

Winter Examination 1999

D Pharm First Year

Health Education and Community Pharmacy

Q 1. Answer any *five* of the following:

a. Define the term health. State the dimensions of health.
b. State the objectives of family planning.

c. What are surface infections?
d. State any four natural methods of contraception.
e. Define the term mortality and morbidity.
f. What is balanced diet?
g. Fill in the blanks:
   i. Deficiency of thiamine results in ________.
   ii. Marasmus disease is caused due to deficiency of ________.
   iii. Hemochromatosis is caused due to excessive storage of ________.
   iv. ________ is a condition caused due to deficiency of vitamin A.

Q 2. Answer any *four* of the following:

a. What is mental health? State major types of mental disorders.
b. What are proteins? State the functions of proteins.
c. Name the determinants of health.
d. Define the term 'demography'. State the various stages of demographic cycle.
e. Describe the emergency treatment in cause of shock.
f. Write a note on slow and filter.

Q 3. Answer any *four* of the following:

a. What is fertility? Discuss in brief the factors affecting fertility.
b. What are the methods of artificial respiration? Explain mouth to mouth resuscitation.
c. Define the term noise. State the ill-effects of noise.
d. Discuss the design and mechanism of septic tank.
e. Give the classification of bacteria on the basis of shape and arrangement.
f. Write a note on prevention and control of cancer.

Q 4. Answer any *four* of the following:

a. Discuss the various modes of transmission of communicable diseases.
b. Give the method and importance of gram staining.
c. What are insecticides and pesticides? Give the classification of insecticides with suitable examples.
d. What are the sources of water pollution? How water pollution can be prevented?
e. What is hydrophobia? Give the causative agent, mode of transmission and symptoms for hydrophobia.
f. What is diabetes mellitus? State the causes for diabetes.

Q 5. Answer any *four* of the following:

a. State the uses of epidemiology.
b. What is isolation? What care should be taken in house isolation or in siolation at home?
c. What is hypertension? What are the predisposing factors for hypertension? State its complications.
d. Differentiate between hepatitis "A" and hepatitis "B" infection.
e. Give the causative agent, mode of transmission and control for tuberculosis.
f. What are fungi? Give the systematic calssification of fungi.

Q 6. Answer any *four* of the following:

a. Write a note on AIDS.
b. What is ventilation? State the various types of ventilation. Give the uses of ventilation.
c. Write a note on IUDs.
d. Classify minerals. State the functions of minerals.
e. Discuss in brief the various nutrition related programmes developed by government of India.
f. Explain in short elements of minor surgery and dressing.

Summer Examination 2000

D Pharm First Year

Health Education and Community Pharmacy

Q 1. Answer any *five* of the following:

a. What are minerals? How will you classify them?
b. State the important functions of food.
c. Give the causative agent and symptoms of whooping cough.
d. State two ifectious diseases each carried by insects:
   i. House fly ii. Sand fly
e. State the ill-effects of noise.
f. What are stains and dyes? State the purpose of staining.
g. Give the mechanism of chlorination of water.

Q 2. Answer any *four* of the following:

a. Define the term mental health. Discuss in brief the major types of mental disorders.
b. What are zoonotic diseases? Classify them with examples.
c. What are essential amino acids? Name them.
d. What is fertility? State the factors affecting fertility.

e. Define the term first aid? State the major principles of first aid.
f. What are the sources of water pollution? How water pollution can be prevented?

Q 3. Answer any *four* of the following:

a. State the types and uses of ventilation.
b. State the classification of bacteria on the basis of shape and arrangements.
c. Define the term health. Name the indicators used for the assessment of health.
d. What is kwashiorkor disease? Give its symptoms and mode of treatment.
e. What are hormonal contraceptives? State their advantages and disadvantages.
f. Describe the general first aid treatment for fractures.

Q 4. Answer any *four* of the following:

a. Explain the process of purification of water on a large scale by slow sand filter with a well-labelled diagram.
b. What are fungi? Give the systematic classification of fungi.
c. What is diabetes? State the types, and causes for diabetes.
d. What is epidemiology? Give the uses of epidemiology.
e. State how the pharmacist can promote family planning.
f. What do you mean by hydrophodia? How it is caused? Give its prevention and control.

Q 5. Answer any *four* of the following:

a. State and explain the concepts of prevention of diseases.
b. Define the term immunity and immunization.
c. Describe the various methods for isolation of bacteria.
d. Define the term "demography". Explain in brief the various stages of demographic cycle.
e. State the differet forms of beriberi. Discuss any one of them.
f. Describe the methods for disposal of refuse.

Q 6. Answer any *four* of the following:

a. Give the causative agent symptoms and preventive measures for malaria.
b. What are nosocomial infections? State the factors responsible for nosocomial infections.
c. Explain the causes of night blindness. Discuss its prevention and treatment.
d. Give the method and importance of Gram staining.

e. Discuss the disinfection procedure for infected:
   i. Stools   ii. Sputum
f. Write a note on botulism.

Winter Examination 2000

D Pharm First Year

Health Education and Community Pharmacy

Q 1. Answer any *five* of the following:

a. Define the term health. State the dimensions of health.
b. State the functions of minerals.
c. Give the advantages of chlorination of water.
d. What is sewage? What are the aims of sewage treatment.
e. What are splints? State the various types of splints.
f. Define the term incidence and prevalence.
g. State the ill effects of noise.

Q 2. Answer any *four* of the following:

a. What is disease? What are the concepts of prevention of diseases?
b. State the different methods of artificial respiration. Explain Holger-Nielsen method.
c. Classify family planning methods with example.
d. Describe the first aid treatment for burns.
e. State the factors which determine good lighting. How best utilisation of day light can be done?
f. State the various methods for isolation of bacteria.

Q 3. Answer any *four* of the following:

a. Describe in brief the major types of fungal diseases.
b. Give the method and importance of gram staining.
c. Describe the general first aid treatment for fractures.
d. Give the causative agent, mode of transmission and symptoms of thyroid.
e. What is coronary heart disease? State the forms and predisposing factors for CHD.
f. Name the types of eipdemiology methods. Describe analytical epidemiology.

Q 4. Answer any *four* of the following:

a. Name the glands and hormones which plays important role in reproduction.

b. What do you mean by determinants of health? State various factors which determin health.
c. What is balanced diet? What are the common deficiencies in Indian diet.
d. Explain in short the elements of minor surgery and dressings.
e. What is food poisoning? State its types and the preventive measures.
f. What is shock? Describe the first aid treatment for shock.

Q 5. Answer any *four* of the following:

a. What are fungi? Give the systematic classification of fungi.
b. Describe different clinical forms of leprosy.
c. Explain the process of purification of water on large scale by rapid sand filter.
d. What are proteins? State the functions of proteins.
e. Discuss the design and mechanism of septic tank.
f. Give the causative agent, symptoms and preventive measures for malaria.

Q 6. Answer any *four* of the following:

a. State the different forms of beriberi. Discuss any one of them.
b. Give the causative organism, mode of transmission and symptoms of tuberculosis.
c. State the sources and functions of vitamin C.
d. Discuss the various types of disinfection methods.
e. Enlist the various arthropods and diseases transmitted by them.
f. State the role of pharmacist in family planning.

Summer Examination 2001

D Pharm First Year

Health Education and Community Pharmacy

Q 1. Answer any *five* of the following:

a. State the factors affecting fertility.
b. Define the term endemic and epidemic.
c. Give the composition of air. State its importance.
d. What do the following abbreviations stand for:

i. BCG	iii. STD
ii. AIDS	iv. DPT

e. Define the term microbiology.
f. What is benign tumour and malignant tumour?
g. State the causative agents and symptoms of diphtheria.
h. Give the advantages and disadvantages of condom.

Q 2. Answer any *four* of the following:

a. Discuss the concept of prevention of diseases.
b. What are stains and dyes? State the purpose of staining.
c. What are the sources of water pollution? How water pollution can be prevented?
d. What are essential amino acids? Name them.
e. Name the indicators used for the assessment of health.
f. State how pharmacist can promote family planning.

Q 3. Solve any *four* of the following:

a. What are insecticides? Give the calssification of insecticides.
b. What is sewage and sullage? What are the aims of sewage treatment?
c. Describe the emergency treatment in case of burns.
d. What is diabetes? State its types and causes.
e. Give the causative agent, mode of transmission, and symptoms of measles.
f. What are splints? What are the different types of splints?

Q 4. Answer any *four* of the following:

a. What are fats? Give the sources and functions of fats.
b. Write a note on hormonal contraceptives.
c. State the different types of hepatitis with causative agents. Give the symptoms, mode of transmission and control of hepatitis-A.
d. Give the method and importance of acid-fast staining.
e. Give the causative organism, symptoms, mode of transmission for malaria.
f. What is disinfection? What are the types of disinfection.

Q 5. Solve any *four* of the following:

a. Define the term viruses. Classify them with examples.
b. What are zoonotic diseases? Classify them with examples.
c. Disucuss in brief the major types of mental disorders.
d. What is shock? Describe the first aid treatment in shock.
e. State the different methods for isolation of bacteria. Discuss any one.
f. Define the term immunity. Elaborate different components of immune system.

Q 6. Answer any *four* of the following:

a. Write a note on kwashiorkor disease.
b. State and discuss the methods for small scale purification of water.
c. State the natural methods of contraception. Explain coitus interruptus.
d. Describe different clinical forms of leprosy.

e. Explain the cause of night blindness. Discuss its prevention and treatment.
f. Elaborate the sources and types of hospital acquired infection.

Winter Examination 2001

D Pharm First Year

Health Education and Community Pharmacy

Q 1. Answer any *five* of the following:

a. State the purpose of staining the microorganisms.
b. Define the term disinfection and disinfectant.
c. State the disinfection procedure for infected faeces.
d. What do the following abbreviations stand for:
   i. STD
   ii. DPT
   iii. BCG
   iv. AIDS
e. What is scurvy? What is it due to?
f. Define the term incidence and prevalence.
g. Give the advantages and disadvantages of condom.
h. State the functions of proteins.

Q 2. Answer any *four* of the following:

a. What are fungi? Give the systematic classification of fungi.
b. Describe different clinical forms of leprosy.
c. Write a note on rapid sand filter.
d. What is hardness of water? What are the disadvantages of hard water?
e. What is benign tumour and malignant tumour? State the various causes of cancer.
f. Define the term health. Discuss in brief the various dimensions of health.
g. Write a note on disposal of solid waste.

Q 3. Solve any *four* of the following:

a. Name the types of epidemiology methods. Describe analytical epidemiology.
b. Write a note on intrauterine devices (IUD).
c. Classify minerals. State the functions of minerals.
d. Define the term immunity. Elaborate different components of immune system.
e. Write a note on Wilson's disease.
f. What are the methods of artificial respiration? Explain kiss of life.
g. What is coronary heart disease? State the form and predisposing factors for CHD.

Q 4. Solve any *four* of the following:

a. Write a note on botulism.
b. Discuss the design and mechanism of septic tank.
c. What is virus? Give the calssification of virus with example.
d. Give the classification of family planning methods with example.
e. Give the causative agent, symptoms and mode of transmission of diphtheria.
f. What is balanced diet? What are the common deficiencies in Indian diet?

Q 5. Answer any *four* of the following:

a. Define the term "medical entomology". Give the examples of arthropods and the diseases spread by them.
b. What are the causes of blindness? Suggest measures necessary for its prevention.
c. What are different types of immunizing agents? Define and classify vaccines.
d. Give the causative agent, symptoms, prevention and control of poliomyelitis.
e. What are hospital acquired infections? State the sources and types of hospital acquired infections.
f. State and discuss the methods for small scale purification of water.

Q 6. Solve any *four* of the following:

a. What is sewage and sullage? What are the aims of sewage treatment?
b. Describe the emergency treatment in case of burns.
c. What are zoonotic diseases? Classify them with examples.
d. State the different types of hepatitis with causative agent, give the symptoms, mode of transmission and control of hepatitis-B.
e. What is shock? Describe the first aid treatment in shock.
f. Name the glands and hormones with their role in reproduction.
g. Write a short note on population explosion in India.

Summer Examination 2002

D Pharm First Year

Health Education and Community Pharmacy

Q 1. Answer any *five* of the following:

a. Name the causative agent of following diseases (any *two*):

i. Diphtheria
ii. Typhoid
iii. Food poisoning

b. i. Name one food borne disease.
   ii. Name on arthropod borne disease.

c. Name the disease caused due to deficiency of:
   i. Vitamin D.
   ii. Vitamin K

d. What are different methods of transmission of disease?

e. Match the following:

i. Fluorine	1. Hypothyroidism
ii. Iodine	2. Dental caries
iii. Iron	3. Haemophilia
iv. Zinc	4. Skin disorders
	5. Anaemia

f. Define the terms:
   i. Microbiology
   ii. Balanced diet

Q 2. Answer any *four* of the following:

a. Classify food with examples.
b. Define health. What are its indicators?
c. Write a note on "natural history of diseases".
d. What are the sources and functions of proteins?
e. What are the national programmes related to nutrition developed by government of India?
f. Give the causative agent, mode of transmission and treatment for "whooping cough".

Q 3. Answer any *four* of the following:

a. Give the advantages and disadvantages of IUD.
b. What is demography? Explain demographic cycle.
c. Explain role of pharmacist in promoting family planning.
d. Explain Holger-Nielsen method of artificial respiration.
e. What are different family planning methods?
f. Give the first aid treatment for burns.

Q 4. Answer any *four* of the following:

a. State main source of water supply.
b. State the ill-effects of light on the body.
c. Name any three airborne diseases.
d. Write a note on "streak plate" technique.
e. What is acid fast staining? Describe it.
f. Give causative agent, mode of transmission and symptoms of "measles".

Q 5. Answer any *four* of the following:

a. What are the causes and preventive measures for "diabetes"?

b. Define:

i. Epidemic disease

ii. Endemic disease

iii. Pandemic disease

c. Write a note on "immunization schedule".

d. Give the causes for blindness.

e. Give the disinfection procedure for faeces and dead bodies.

f. Classify disinfectants with examples.

Q 6. Give the causative agent, mode of transmission and treatment of any *four* of the following diseases.

a. Cholera

b. TB

c. AIDS

d. Rabies

e. Malaria

f. Plague

Winter Examination 2002

D Pharm First Year

Health Education and Community Pharmacy

Q 1. Answer any *five* of the following:

a. Name the causative agent of following diseases (any *two*):

i. Poliomyelitis

ii. Cholera

iii. Measles

b. i. Name one airborne disease.

ii. Name one waterborne disease.

c. Define the terms:

i. Epidemiology

ii. Demography

d. What are different methods of transmission of disease?

e. Name the disease caused due to deficiency of:

i. Vitamin 'A'

ii. Vitamin 'C'

f. Give the incubation period for:

i. Typhoid

ii. Smallpox

iii. Influenza

Q 2. Answer any *four* of the following:

a. Describe various aspects of health.
b. Define health. What are its determinants?
c. Write a note on "economic cycle of disease".
d. What are the sources and functions for proteins?
e. What are the national programmes related to nutrition developed by government of India?
f. Give the causative agent, mode of transmission and treatment for diphtheria.

Q 3. Answer any *four* of the following:

a. Give the advantages and disadvantages of condom.
b. What are the major principles of "first aid".
c. Explain the role of pharmacist in promoting family planning.
d. Explain silvesters method of artificial respiration.
e. What are the different family planning methods?
f. Give the first aid treatment of snake bite.

Q 4. Answer any *four* of the following:

a. State the main sources of water supply.
b. State the ill-effects of noise.
c. Name any three arthropod borne diseases and give the life cycle of any one.
d. Write a note on "pour plate technique".
e. What is "Gram staining"? Describe it.
f. Give the causative agent, mode of transmission and symptoms of chickenpox.

Q 5. Answer any *four* of the following:

a. What are the causes and preventive measures for CHD?
b. Define:
   i. Epidemic disease
   ii. Endemic disease
   iii. Pandemic disease
c. Write a note on "immunization schedule".
d. Give the causes for cancer.
e. Give the disinfection procedure for sputum and urine.
f. Classify disinfectants with examples.

Q 6. Give the causative agent, mode of transmission, prevention and treatment of the following diseases (any *four*):

a. TB
b. Hepatitis

c. Typhoid
d. Malaria
e. Leprosy
f. Syphilis

Summer Examination 2003

D Pharm First Year

Health Education and Community Pharmacy

Q 1. Answer any *five* of the following:

a. Define the terms:
   i. Vectors ii. Formites
b. Name the causative agent for following disease:
   i. Pertusis ii. Enteric fever
c. What are the various sources of water?
d. Name two airborne and two waterborne diseases.
e. What is epidemic and endemic disease?
f. What is the composition of ORS?
g. Give the composition of balanced diet.

Q 2. Answer any *three* of the following:

a. Define the terms:
   i. Physical health iii. Social health
   ii. Mental health iv. Family welfare
b. Describe the various determinants of health.
c. Explain the concept of prevention of disease.
d. Give the deficiency diseases of fat soluble vitamins.
e. Discuss the functions of minerals in the body.

Q 3. Answer any *four* of the following:

a. Describe in brief about population problem in India.
b. How will you provide first aid treatment for snake bite.
c. Describe Holger-Nielsen method of artificial respiration.
d. What is sewage? Describe one method of sewage treatment.
e. Define shock. Mention different types of shock. Describe first aid treatment for it.
f. What is air pollution? Mention its causes and preventive measures.

Q 4. Answer any *four* of the following:

a. Define demography. Describe the demographic cycle.
b. Describe in brief the house-hold methods of purification of water.

c. Describe natural methods of family planning.
d. Write a note on "national immunization schedule".
e. Give the disinfections procedures for following:
   i. Faeces and urine ii. Dead bodies
f. Define the terms:
   i. Communicable disease iii. First aid
   ii. Vaccines iv. Pandemic

Q 5. Tabulate the information of causative agent, modes of transmission, symptoms and prevention of any *four* of the following:

a. Malaria
b. Hepatitis B
c. Plague
d. Tetanus
e. Syphilis
f. Trachoma

Q 6. Answer any *four* of the following:

a. With the help of neat labelled diagram describe the structure of bacteria.
b. Name the various techniques used for isolation of bacteria. Describe any one.
c. Give the procedure of acid fast staining.
d. Give the types and causes of diabetes mellitus.
e. Write a note on food poisoning.
f. Describe prevention and control of blindness.

Winter Examination 2003

D Pharm First Year

Health Education and Community Pharmacy

Q 1. Answer any *five* of the following:

a. Define the terms:
   i. Incubation period
   ii. Microbiology
b. Name the causative agent for following disease.
   i. Syphilis
   ii. Cholera
c. Differentiate between active and passive immunity.

d. Name two diseases each of:
   i. Sexually transmitted disease
   ii. Noncommunicable diseases
e. What is antiseptic and disinfectant?
f. What are different methods of transmission of disease?
g. Describe cold chain storage of vaccines.

Q 2. Answer any *three* of the following:

a. Mention the vector for following diseases.
   i. Kala azar
   ii. Trypanosomiasis
   iii. Malaria
   iv. Plague
b. Describe various indicators of health.
c. Write a note on "epidemiological triad".
d. Describe the uses and deficiency diseases of proteins.
e. Give the deficiency diseases of vitamin B complex.

Q 3. Answer any *four* of the following:

a. Write in brief about 'slow sand filter'.
b. Write a note on 'noise pollution'.
c. Describe Silvester method of artificial respiration.
d. What is fracture? Give its types. Describe general first aid measures for it.
e. Name various heart diseases. Describe first aid treatment for any one.
f. Define first aid. Give its principles.

Q 4. Answer any *four* of the following:

a. Define epidemiology. Describe its uses.
b. Describe in brief the methods of solid, waste disposal.
c. Write a note on "hospital acquired infections".
d. Describe permanent methods of family planning.
e. Give disinfection procedures for following:
   i. Sputum
   ii. Rooms
f. Define the terms:
   i. Medical entomology
   ii. Toxoids
   iii. Epidemic
   iv. Sporadic

Q 5. Tabulate the information of causative agent, modes of transmission, symptoms and prevention of any four of the following:

a. Tuberculosis
b. Typhoid
c. Diphtheria
d. Leprosy
e. Chickenpox
f. Filariasis

Q 6. Answer any *four* of the following:

a. Classify bacteria on the basis of their shape and arrangement.
b. Write in brief about 'hormonal contraceptives".
c. Write a note on "fungal infections".
d. Give the types and causes of hypertension.
e. Mention types of cancer and write its causes.
f. Describe the prevention and control of diabetes.

Summer Examination 2004

D Pharm First Year

Health Education and Community Pharmacy

Q 1. Attempt any *five* of the following:

a. Name the causative agent of following diseases.
   i. Cholera
   ii. Diphtheria
   iii. Chickenpox
   iv. Measles
b. Give two examples of each:
   i. Air-borne diseases
   ii. Water-borne diseases
   iii. Arthropod-borne diseases
   iv. Surface infections
c. Define the terms:
   i. Epidemiology
   ii. Demography
   iii. Microbiology
   iv. Balanced diet
d. What do you know about:
   i. Physical health
   ii. Mental health
   iii. Social health
   iv. Spiritual health
e. Name the disease caused due to deficiency of:
   i. Vitamin A
   ii. Vitamin D
   iii. Vitamin C
   iv. Vitamin B_{12}
f. Define the terms:
   i. Antiseptic and disinfectant
   ii. Active and passive immunity

g. What do you know about:
   i. Exotoxin and endotoxin
   ii. Vasectomy and tubectomy

Q 2. Attempt any *four* of the following:

a. Describe the various determinants of health.
b. Explain the concept of prevention of disease.
c. Explain with flow diagram "economic cycle of a disease".
d. Give a brief account of calcium and iron.
e. What are the mortality indicators of health?
f. Describe the various causative agents of a disease.

Q 3. Attempt any *four* of the following:

a. Define first aid. Give its major principles.
b. Explain "back pressure arm lift" method.
c. Describe the 'first aid' for burns.
d. What is fracture? Give its type. What first aid would you give in fracture?
e. Describe the chemical methods of water purification.
f. Name the various methods of solid waste disposal. Explain any one.

Q 4. Attempt any *four* of the following:

a. With a labelled diagram describe the structure of bacteria.
b. Write a note on "Gram's staining method".
c. Define contraceptives. Enlist the various contraceptive methods.
d. Give the advantages and disadvantages of oral contraceptives.
e. Describe in short "rhythm method" of contraception.
f. Describe "streak plate" method.

Q 5. Attempt any *four* of the following:

a. Give the prevention and control of cancer.
b. Describe the causes, prevention and control of hypertension.
c. Give the types, symptoms and causes of diabetes.
d. What are nosocomial infections? Describe prevention and control of a nosocomial infection.
e. Write a note on "national immunization schedule".
f. Give any two methods each for disinfection of sputum and dead bodies.

Q 6. Give the causative agent, mode of transmission and prevention of any *four* of the following:

a. TB
b. Poliomyelitis
c. Malaria
d. Tetanus
e. Syphilis
f. AIDS

Winter Examination 2004

D Pharm First Year

Health Education and Community Pharmacy

Q 1. Attempt any *five* of the following:

a. Name the causative agent of following diseases.
   i. Typhoid
   ii. AIDS
   iii. Hepatitis
   iv. Amoebiasis

b. Give two examples of each:
   i. Chemical disinfection methods
   ii. Water borne diseases
   iii. Sources of water supply
   iv. Temporary contraceptive methods

c. Define the terms:
   i. Immunity
   ii. Diabetes mellitus
   iii. Air pollution
   iv. Nutrition

d. What do you know about:
   i. Haemoglobin
   ii. Conjunctivitis
   iii. Aspiration
   iv. Mast cell

e. Name the disease caused due to deficiency of:
   i. Copper
   ii. Iodine
   iii. Fluorine
   iv. Iron

f. Define the terms:
   i. Vaccines
   ii. Bacteria

g. What do you know about:
   i. WHO
   ii. Red Cross

Q 2. Attempt any *four* of the following:

a. Define health. Discuss morality indicators.
b. What is haemorrhage? Explain the process of coagulations.
c. Describe the various diseases caused by arthropods.
d. Explain definition, types and growth characters of 'fungi'.
e. What is cancer? Discuss its primary prevention.
f. Discusss in detail types of immunoglobulins.

Q 3. Attempt any *four* of the following:

a. Chart out the national immunization schedule.
b. Define coronary heart disease. Discuss the primary prevention.
c. Discuss in detail 'noise pollution'.
d. Define burns. Explain first aid treatment of burns.
e. What is family planning? Describe its benefits.
f. Define vitamins. Thoroughly discuss 'water soluble vitamins'.

Q 4. Attempt any *four* of the following:

a. Discuss in detail 'concept of disease'.
b. Explain different staining techniques for the study of bacteria.
c. Describe commonly used antiseptics for dressings.
d. Define blindness. Discuss causes and prevention of blindness.
e. Describe various methods of water purification.
f. Explain the importance of breastfeeding.

Q 5. Attempt any *four* of the following:

a. What is a fracture? Explain types, signs, symptoms and first aid for it.
b. Discuss the role of pharmacist in community.
c. What is disinfection? Describe all the methods of disinfection.
d. Define 'food', classify foods and discuss the hazards of malnutrition.
e. What are the types of sutures? Discuss points to remember in suture technique.
f. Explain in detail cardiopulmonary resuscitation.

Q 6. Give the causative agent, mode of transmission and prevention of any *four* of the following:

a. Syphilis
b. Leprosy
c. Malaria
d. Poliomyelitis
e. Ascariasis
f. Tuberculosis

Summer Examination 2005

D Pharm First Year

Health Education and Community Pharmacy

Q 1. Attempt any *five* of the following:

a. What is health? Mention various dimension of health.
b. What is disease? Give natural history of disease.
c. Classify minerals. Discuss importance of iodine in the body.
d. Give composition of air. How it differs from polluted air?
e. What is fracture? Give its types.
f. Differentiate between communicable and noncommunicable diseases with example.
g. Define the following terms:
   i. Immunization   ii. Vaccine

Q 2. Answer any *four* of the following:

a. What are health determinants? Explain in brief.
b. What are the concepts of prevention of diseases?
c. Give sources of food with their dietary importance.
d. Write various steps of slow sand filtration for water purification.
e. Explain demographic cycle and comment on it.
f. What is immunity? Explain active and passive immunity.

Q 3. Answer any *four* of the following:

a. Discuss health indicators with their role in determination of health.
b. What is vitamin? Explain function of vitamins A and C.
c. What is stain? Explain various stains with their use in staining techniques.
d. Discuss about diseases caused by proteins.
e. What is poisoning? Give types of poisoning with first aid treatment.
f. Explain types of cancer. Give the factors responsible for cancer.

Q 4. Answer any *four* of the following:

a. What are carbohydrates? Give their sources with examples.
b. Explain sources of water with examples.
c. What is shock? Explain in with first aid treatment.
d. Explain different methods of family planning.
e. What is epidemiology? Give its importance to the society.
f. Give long forms of the following with brief explanation:
   i. RTI
   ii. UTI
   iii. STD
   iv. CHD
   v. DPT
   vi. MMR
   vii. HIV

Q 5. Answer any *four* of the following:

a. What is microbiology? Give its importance.
b. What do you mean by industrial air pollution? How it affects human life?
c. What is artificial respiration? Explain mouth to nose respiration.
d. Differentiate between malaria and filaria according to their causative agents, vectors, symptoms and preventive measures.
e. Give disinfection procedures for the following:
   i. Sputum
   ii. Room
   iii. Instuments
f. Discuss in detail noise pollution.

Q 6. Answer any *four* of the following:

a. Give classification of bacteria according to its size and shape.
b. What is water pollution? Give its impact on human life.
c. Explain briefly different methods of solid waste disposal.
d. Explain national policy of family planning with its importance.
e. What is AIDS? Explain it in brief.
f. What is diabetes? Give its severity in India and steps to control it.

Winter Examination 2005

D Pharm First Year

Health Education and Community Pharmacy

Q 1. Attempt any *five* of the following:

a. Define the terms:
   i. Health
   ii. Disease
   iii. Epidemic
   iv. First aid
b. What do you know about:
   i. Family planning
   ii. Family welfare
   iii. Demography
   iv. Balanced diet
c. Name the disease due to the following causative agent:
   i. *Bordetella pertussis*
   ii. Varicella-zoster
   iii. *Entamoeba histolytica*
   iv. *Yersinia pestis*
d. Give two examples of each:
   i. Zoonotic diseases
   ii. Respiratory infections
   iii. Intestinal infections
   iv. STDs
e. Name the vitamin causing the following deficiency disease.
   i. Xerophthalmia
   ii. Rickets
   iii. Megaloblastic anaemia
   iv. Beriberi
f. What do you know about:
   i. Shapte of bacteria
   ii. Types of fungi
g. Explain the terms:
   i. Hypertension
   ii. Stroke
   iii. Diabetes mellitus
   iv. Cancer

Q 2. Attempt any *four* of the following:

a. Explain the dimensions of health.
b. Explain natural history of disease and its phases.
c. Name various indicators used for measurement of health status and explain any two.

d. Name the protein deficiency diseases and explain how it can be prevented?
e. Give the functions of foods. Give role of calcium in body.
f. Write various steps of rapid sand filtration for purifications of water.

Q 3. Attempt any *four* of the following:

a. Elaborate various stages of demographic cycle.
b. Write effect of noise pollution.
c. Give the various sources of water and explain how water can be contaminated?
d. What are contraceptives? Name some temporary methods and some permanent methods of contraception.
e. Explain first aid for snake poisoning.
f. Explain household methods of water purification.

Q 4. Attempt any *four* of the following:

a. Draw a neat labelled diagram of structure of a typical virus.
b. Give causative agent, mode of transmission and prevention of AIDS.
c. Give the cause and preventive measures for hypertension.
d. Give the various techniques for isolation of microorganisms.
e. Mention the types of hepatitis, give the causative organisms and modes of transmission.
f. What are the types of diabetes? How can diabetes be controlled?

Q 5. Attempt any *four* of the following:

a. What is epidemiology? What are its methods?
b. What is disinfection? Give its types.
c. Give the "National Immunization Schedule".
d. What is sewage? Explain biological treatment of sewage.
e. What are condoms? What are its advantages and disadvantages?
f. What is benign tumour and malignant tumour? Give causes of cancer.

Q 6. Attempt any *four* of the following:

a. What are the functions of proteins?
b. Give the importance of vitamin A, and it's deficiency diseases.
c. Give the first aid for fracture.
d. Give the causative agent, mode of transmission and prevention of malaria.
e. Classify microorganisms.
f. Give the causative agent, mode of transmission and prevention of tuberculosis.

Summer Examination 2006

D Pharm First Year

Health Education and Community Pharmacy

Q 1. Attempt any *five* of the following:

a. Define the term:
   i. Health
   ii. Disease
   iii. Demography
   iv. Family planning

b. Explain the term:
   i. Incubation period
   ii. Contraceptive
   iii. First aid
   iv. Entamology

c. Give the mode of transmission of:
   i. Tuberculosis
   ii. Cholera
   iii. Malaria
   iv. Syphilis

d. Give the long forms of following abbreviations:
   i. AIDS
   ii. STD
   iii. IUD
   iv. WHO

e. Name a vitamin given in the treatment of following deficiency diseases/disorders.
   i. Pellagra
   ii. Scurvy
   iii. Beriberi
   iv. Pernicious anaemia

f. Compare the following:
   i. Gram +ve and Gram –ve bacteria
   ii. RNA and DNA virus

g. Elaborate the following terms:
   i. Epidemic
   ii. Pandemic
   iii. Contagious
   iv. Zoonosis

Q 2. Attempt any *four* of the following:

a. Name various dimensions of health. Elaborate any one in detail.
b. Explain the "natural history of the diseases".
c. What are proteins. Name and describe protein malnutrition diseases.
d. What is disease agent. Classify them with examples.
e. Give the sources and function of vitamin D.
f. Classify minerals with examples. Explain the role of iodine.

Q 3. Attempt any *four* of the following:

a. Classify contraceptive methods with examples.
b. Describe vasectomy or tubectomy method.
c. What are the objectives achieved by a family planning.
d. Write a note on elements of minory surgery.

e. Describe the first aid treatment for snake bite.
f. Define fertility and discuss various factors affecting fertility.

Q 4. Attempt any *four* of the following:

a. Describe with a flow diagram 'rapid sand filter".
b. Write a note on "isolation of pure culture".
c. Give composition of air. How the air is polluted?
d. Name any four arthropods with disease transmitted by them.
e. Classify bacteria depending upon their shape.
f. What is the need for staining? Describe "Ziehl-Neelsen method".

Q 5. Attept any *four* of the following:

a. What is the cause of diabetes mellitus. How it is prevented.
b. Give different types of cancer. How it can be prevented.
c. Write a note on DPT.
d. What are noncommunicable disease. Give the four causes of non-communicable diseases.
e. Give the prevention and treatment of hypertension.
f. Define disinfection. Describe disinfection procedure for sputum and linen.

Q 6. Tabulate the following by giving causative agent, mode of transmission and prevention (any *four*):

a. AIDS
b. Leprosy
c. Rabies
d. Plague
e. Polio
f. Chickenpox

Winter Examination 2006

D Pharm First Year

Health Education and Community Pharmacy

Q 1. Attempt any *four* of the following:

a. Define the terms:
   i. Incubation period
   ii. Mortality
   iii. Poison
   iv. Shock
   v. Vaccines

b. Name the causative agent of the following diseases:
   i. Tuberculosis
   ii. Cholera
   iii. Chickenpox
   iv. Malaria
   v. Rabies

c. Give long form of the following with brief explanation.
   i. WHO
   ii. BCG
   iii. TT
   iv. ORS
   v. STD

d. Give diseases occurring due to deficiency of:
   i. Vitamin A
   ii. Vitamin D
   iii. Vitamin C
   iv. Vitamin K
   v. Folic acid

e. What do you know about:
   i. Immunoglobulins
   ii. Noise pollution
   iii. Trachoma
   iv. Burns
   v. Fungi

f. State important inorganic elements/minerals related to following:
   i. Haemoglobin
   ii. Erythropoiesis
   iii Enlargement of thyroid
   iv. Contraction of muscles
   v. Wilson's disease

Q 2. Answer any *four* of the following:

a. Explain the classification of viruses.
b. What do you know about 'sewage' and its treatment?
c. Describe in detail about hospital acquired infections.
d. Define demography. Discuss problems related to excess population.
e. What is balanced diet? Write about its advantages.
f. Write note on 'cold chain storage of vaccines'.

Q 3. Answer any *four* of the following:

a. Enlist medically important bacterias. What is gram staining?
b. Define first aid. What is its scope and objectives?
c. Discuss the design and mechanism of septic tank.
d. Write short note on hormonal contraceptives.
e. What is air pollution? Discuss its prevention and control.
f. Discuss the role of pharmacist in family planning programme.

Q 4. Answer any *four* of the following:

a. Discuss in detail causative agent, symptoms, transmission, prevention and control of influenza.
b. What is AIDS? Explain its prevention.
c. Give a short note on types of disinfection.
d. Write different modes of transmission of diseases.
e. Define health. Describe the dimensions of health.
f. Explain in detail the various diseases occurring due to the deficiency of vitamin B complex group.

Q 5. Answer any *four* of the following:

a. What are proteins? Explain sources and deficiency of proteins.
b. State types of epidemiology, discuss any one type in details.
c. Write a note on 'food poisoning'.
d. What are the zoonotic disease? Give examples and preventive measures.
e. Discuss the first aid of snake bite.

Q 6. Answer any *four* of the following:

Discuss the causative factors, symptoms and preventive measures of:

a. Diabetes
b. Cancer
c. Syphilis
d. Hypertension
e. Whooping cough
f. Tuberculosis

Summer Examination 2007

D Pharm First Year

Health Education and Community Pharmacy

Q 1. Attempt any *five* of the following:

a. Define the terms 'stains' and state the purposes of staining.
b. Define 'fertility' and state the factors affecting fertility.
c. Name the causative agent of the following disease. (Any *two*)
   i. Plague
   ii. Filariasis
   iii. AIDS
d. What is meant by 'essential amino acids'? Enlist different EAAs.
e. Name one disease each caused due to deficiency (any *two*):
   i. Iodine
   ii. Vitamin B_{12}
   iii. Vitamin D
f. Define the terms (any *two*):
   i. Infection
   ii. Incubation period
   iii. Microbiology
g. Name one disease caused by the following arthropods (any *two*):
   i. House fly
   ii. Mosquito
   iii. Flea

Q 2. Answer any *four* of the following:

a. Define 'health'. Describe briefly various dimensions of health.
b. Describe 'national immunization schedule'.
c. Name different 'host defence mechanisms' working in our body. Differentiate between active and passive immunity.

d. Define 'staining'. Classify the staining procedures used for the microorganisms. Give details of Gram's staining.
e. What are 'hospital acquired infections'? State some common types of such infections and the control measures to be taken to prevent them.
f. Define 'disinfection'. Give recommended distinction procedure for faeces and urine.

Q 3. Answer any *four* of the following:

a. What is meant by 'isolation of pure culture? Enlist different methods used for isolation of bacteria.
b. What is meant by 'determinants of health'? Classify them and explain how socioeconomic conditions act as health determinants.
c. Define 'epidemiology'. What are the uses of epidemiology?
d. What is 'hydrophobia'? Why is it so named? Give causative agent, symptoms and prevention of hydrophobia.
e. Describe cardiopulmonary resuscitation.
f. Classify vitamins. Write sources of vitamin C and vitamin D.

Q 4. Answer any *four* of the following:

a. State different types of epidemiological studies. Explain briefly 'descriptive epidemiology'.
b. Explain different modes of transmission of communicable diseases, examplifying you answer with suitable diseases.
c. What are burns and scalds? Give first aid treatment for burns and scalds.
d. Classify the methods of contraception. Describe different types of Intrauterine Devices (IUDs).
e. Define and describe 'natural history of disease'.
f. What is hypertension? Give causes, preventive measures and treatment of hypertension.

Q 5. Answer any *four* of the following:

a. Draw a well labelled diagram of a bacterial cell. Also calssify bacteria based on their shape and arrangement.
b. Define 'case and 'carrier' of infection. Classify carriers giving suitable examples.
c. Classify and describe various immunological products giving suitable examples.
d. Give details of 'rapid sand filteration' for purification of water.
e. State and explain different types of arrhythmias.
f. Define 'solid wastes'. Explain briefly different methods of solid waste disposal.

Q 6. Answer any *four* of the following:

a. State and explain different types of fungal diseases.
b. Give the causative agent, modes of transmission and preventive measures for diphtheria.
c. Describe general structural features of viruses with the help of a well labelled diagram.
d. What are proteins? Discuss the diseases induced by deficiency of proteins.
e. What is a 'communicable disease'? Name one each of the following:
   i. Arthropod borne infection
   ii. Respiratory tract infection
   iii. Surface infection
   iv. Intestinal infection
   v. Sexually transmitted infection
f. Define 'prevention of disease' and explain the concepts of prevention of diseases.

Winter Examination 2007

D Pharm First Year

Health Education and Community Pharmacy

Q 1. Solve any *five* of the following:

a. Define the terms:
   i. First aid
   ii. Contraceptives
   iii. Zoonotic diseases
   iv. Microbiology
b. Name the disease due to following causative agent:
   i. Varicella-zoster
   ii. *Clostridium tetani*
   iii. *Bordetella pertusis*
   iv. *Yersinia pestis*
c. Name the disease caused due to deficiency of:
   i. Vitamin A
   ii. Vitamin D
   iii. Vitamin C
   iv. Vitamin B_{12}
d. Explain the terms:
   i. Nosocomial infections
   ii. Epidemiology
   iii. Noncommunicable diseases
   iv. Health education
e. Give two examples of each:
   i. Arthropod borne diseases
   ii. Fungal diseases
   iii. Intrauterine devices
   iv. Vaccine

f. What do you know about:
   i. Disinfectant
   ii. Immunity
   iii. Hydrophobia
   iv. Water borne diseases

g. Give the long forms of following abbreviations:
   i. BCG
   ii. DPT
   iii. ORS
   iv. IUD

Q 2. Answer any *four* of the following:

a. What is diabetes mellitus? State the types and causes for diabetes.
b. What are hospital acquired infections? Describe prevention and control of hospital acquired infections.
c. Why the bacteria are stained? Explain the method of gram staining.
d. What is virus? Elaborate major types of viruses and diseases, caused by them.
e. Discuss the disinfection procedure for infected:
   i. Stools
   ii. Sputum
f. What are different sources of water? Give the advantages and disadvantages of any two sources.

Q 3. Answer any *four* of the following:

a. Describe first aid treatment for snake bite.
b. What are methods of artificial respiration? Explain mouth to mouth respiration.
c. What is sewage? What are the aims of sewage treatment?
d. What are the effects of air pollution on health?
e. Explain briefly different methods of solid waste disposal.
f. What is fracture? Describe general first aid for fracture.

Q 4. Answer any *four* of the following:

a. Name the indicators used for assessment of health. Explain any one indicator.
b. What do you mean by natural history of disease? How its knowledge help in the effective treatment of health?
c. State different forms of beriberi. Discuss any one of them.
d. What are essential amino acids? Name them.
e. Give the deficiency disease of iron and calcium.
f. Name the determinants of health.

Q 5. Answer any *four* of the following:

a. Give the classification of bacteria on the basis of shape and arrangement.
b. What is hypertension? What are the causes of hypertension?
c. Differentiate between active and passive immunity.

d. Justify the need of family planning and fertility control.
e. State how the pharmacist can promote family planning.
f. Give the advantages and disadvantages of condom.

Q 6. Give the causative agent, mode of transmission and prevention of any *four* of the following:

a. Tuberculosis
b. AIDS
c. Rabies
d. Typhoid
e. Plague
f. Chickenpox

Summer Examination 2008

D Pharm First Year

Health Education and Community Pharmacy

Q 1. Solve any *five* of the following:

a. Define the terms:
   i. Communicable disease
   ii. Epidemiology
   iii. Health education
   iv. Family planning
b. Name the causative agents of following disease:
   i. Tuberculosis
   ii. Poliomyelitis
   iii. Influenza
   iv. Rabies
c. Give two examples of each:
   i. Water borne diseases
   ii. Arthropod borne disease
   iii. Intestinal infections
   iv. Zoonotic diseases
d. Give the long forms of following abbreviations:
   i. HIV
   ii. DPT
   iii. STD
   iv. IUD
e. Name the diseases caused due to deficiency of:
   i. Vitamin A
   ii. Protein
   iii. Iron
   iv. Iodine
f. What do you know about:
   i. Isolation of patients
   ii. Gram-positive staining of bacteria
g. Give disinfection procedure for:
   i. Urine
   ii. Linen

Q 2. Answer any *four* of the following:

a. Describe various aspects of health.
b. What are proteins? State the functions of proteins.
c. What are hormonal contraceptives? State their advantages and disadvantages.

d. Define first aid. What are the major principles of first aid treatment?
e. What are solid waste? Write in brief the various methods of solid waste disposal.
f. State the various methods of isolation of bacteria. Describe in detail streak plate technique.

Q 3. Answer any *four* of the following:

a. State and explain the concept of prevention of disease.
b. Draw a well labelled diagram of bacterial cell.
c. Give the causative agent, mode of transmission and prevention of leprosy.
d. What is kwashiorkor disease? Give its symptoms and mode of treatment.
e. What is hypertension? Discuss the causative factors, symptoms and prevention of cardiovascular diseases.
f. What are nosocomial infections? Explain the factors responsible for nosocomial infection.

Q 4. Answer any *four* of the following:

a. What is disinfection? Write in detail about any two disinfecting agents.
b. Discuss various methods of arthropod control.
c. Write in detail about principles of prevention and control of communicable diseases.
d. State the different types of hepatitis with causative agents. Give the mode of transmission and control of hepatitis A and hepatitis B.
e. What is the resuscitation method? List out different methods of artificial respiration. Explain in detail Sylvester method.
f. Classify contraceptive methods. Explain about Copper-T and Lippe's loop.

Q 5. Answer any *four* of the following:

a. What is cancer? How it is controlled?
b. What is vitamin? Classify it. Explain functions and deficiency symptoms of vitamin C.
c. Discuss the three indicators used for assessment of health.
d. Describe the first aid treatment for:
   i. Shock
   ii. Burns
e. Explain importance of family planning.
f. Name any four disease transmitted by rodents. Explain in brief how to control rodents.

Q 6. Give the causative agents, mode of transmission and prevention of any *four* of the following:

a. Filariasis
b. Food poisoning
c. Hookworm
d. Tetanus
e. Gonorrhoea
f. Measles

Winter Examination 2008

D Pharm First Year

Health Education and Community Pharmacy

Q 1. Answer the following:

a. Define the terms (any *four*):
   i. Health (According to WHO)
   ii. Sporadic
   iii. Toxoid
   iv. Host
   v. Epidemiology

b. Explain in brief the terms (any *four*):
   i. Chlorine demand
   ii. Mortality
   iii. Contraceptive
   iv. Vaccine
   v. Epidemic

c. Name the causative agent of following diseases (any *four*):
   i. Measles
   ii. Influenza
   iii. Plague
   iv. Smallpox
   v. Whooping cough

d. Give two examples of each (any *four*):
   i. Water borne disease
   ii. Sources of water supply
   iii. Temporary contraceptive methods
   iv. Air borne disease
   v. Antitoxin

e. Give the long forms of following abbreviations (any *four*):
   i. DPT
   ii. STD
   iii. BCG
   iv. ORS
   v. WHO

Q 2. Answer *four* of the following:

a. Explain the various determinant of health.
b. What are essential amino acid? Give its examples.
c. Define demography. Classify family planning methods with example of each.

d. Describe emergency treatment for burns.
e. Enlist the objectives and uses of epidemiology.
f. Write a note on "food poisoning".

Q 3. Answer any *four* of the following:

a. Explain Gram's staining technique.
b. Explain purification of water on large scale.
c. What are proteins? Explain functions and deficiency of proteins.
d. Define disease agent. Classify them with examples.
e. Describe causes and control of diabetes.
f. Explain role of pharmacist in community particularly in nonclinical services.

Q 4. Answer any *four* of the following:

a. Discuss in detail descriptive epidemiology.
b. Explain the design and mechanism of septic tank.
c. Give advantages and disadvantages of condom.
d. State the different forms of beriberi. Describe in brief any one of them.
e. Describe first aid treatment for snakebite.
f. Differentiate between benign and malignant tumours? Enlist factors reponsible for cancer.

Q 5. Answer any *four* of the following:

a. Explain the process of cardiopulmonary resuscitation (CPR).
b. Give in detail principles of disease control and prevention.
c. Describe morphological classification of bacteria.
d. Give the causative agent, symptoms, transmission, prevention and control of tuberculosis.
e. Discuss the demographic cycle. Describe in short one method of permanent contraceptives.
f. Describe effect and control of air pollution.

Q 6. Answer any *four* of the following:

Discuss the causative agents, modes of transmission and preventive measures of:

a. Leprosy
b. Typhoid
c. Polio
d. Gonorrhoea
e. Malaria
f. Rabies

Summer Examination 2009

D Pharm First Year

Health Education and Community Pharmacy

Q 1. Attempt any *two* of the following:

a. Define the terms:
   i. Immunity
   ii. Nutrition
   iii. Microbiology
   iv. Vaccine
   v. Disinfectant

b. Name the causative agent of following diseases:
   i. Filariasis
   ii. Diphtheria
   iii. Hepatitis
   iv. Typhoid
   v. Gonorrhoea

c. Give two examples of each:
   i. Temporary contraceptive methods
   ii. Arthropod borne diseases
   iii. Airborne diseases
   iv. Water borne diseases
   v. Surface infection

Q 2. Answer any *four* of the following:

a. Discuss in detail “concept of disease”.
b. Explain in detail cardiopulmonary resuscitation.
c. What is fracture? Give its type. What first aid would you give in fracture?
d. Define family welfare. Discuss population problems in India.
e. Describe various methods of water purification on large scale.

Q 3. Answer any *four* of the following:

a. Define blindness. Discuss causes and prevention of blindness.
b. Describe the various determinants of health.
c. Write a note on ‘Gram’ staining method.
d. Expalin the types, symptoms and causes of diabetes.
e. Define contraceptives. Describe in short “rhythm method” of contraception.

Q 4. Answer any *four* of the following:

a. Write a note on “national immunization schedule”.
b. What is epidemiology? Write its importance.
c. What is cancer? Explain causes and prevention.
d. Write a note on ‘insect control’.
e. Discuss in detail “air pollution”.

Q 5. Answer any *four* of the following:

a. What is burns? Explain it with first aid treatment.
b. Discuss the role of pharmacist in community health.
c. Describe the causes, prevention and control of hypertension.
d. What are vitamin? Discuss water soluble vitamins.
e. Discuss in detail types of immunoglobulins.

Q 6. Answer any *four* of the following:

a. Describe the structure of bacteria with labelled diagram.
b. What are carbohydrates? Explain sources with examples.
c. Discuss various methods of solid waste disposal.
d. Explain sources of water with examples.
e. What is tuberculosis? Explain its cause symptom and prevention.

Summer Examination 2010

D Pharm First Year

Health Education and Community Pharmacy

Q 1. Attempt any *five* of the following:

a. Define the term:
   i. Health ii. Nutrition
   iii. Incubation period iv. Immunity
b. Give the mode of transmission of:
   i. AIDS ii. Measles
   iii. Amobiasis iv. Trachoma
c. Name a vitamin given in the treatment of following deficiency diseases/disorders:
   i. Bleeding disorders ii. Keratomalacia
   iii. Beriberi iv. Megaloblastic anaemia
d. Give two examples of each:
   i. Natural disinfectants
   ii. Airborne diseases
   iii. Permanent contraceptive methods
   iv. Arthropods borne diseases
e. Compare the following:
   i. Gram +ve and Gram –ve bacteria
   ii. Active immunity and passive immunity
f. Name the causative agent of following diseases:
   i. Chickenpox ii. Plague
   iii. Tuberculosis iv. Rabies

g. What do you know about?
   i. Reservoir
   ii. Antibody
   iii. Cold chain
   iv. Quarantine

Q 2. Attempt any *four* of the following:

a. What is mental health? State major types of metal disorders.
b. Name the various determinants of health and explain in brief.
c. What is kwashiorkar disease? Give its symptoms and mode of treatment.
d. Define the term 'Demography' and explain demographic cycle.
e. Classify contraceptive method with example.
f. What are hormonal contraceptive? How are they classified? Discuss their advantages and disadvantages.

Q 3. Attempt any *four* of the following:

a. Describe the emergency treatment in case of snakebite.
b. What are the general signs and symptoms of fracture? Describe in general, management of fracture.
c. Explain in detail cardio-pulmonary resuscitation (CPR).
d. Define burns. Explain first aid treatment of burns.
e. Explain sources of water with examples.
f. What is hardness of water? What are the disadvantages of hard water?

Q 4. Attempt any *four* of the following:

a. What are air borne diseases? How air borne diseases can be prevented?
b. Write various steps of "slow and filteration" for water purification.
c. Explain briefly different methods of solid waste disposal.
d. What are insecticides? Give the classification of insecticides with examples.
e. Describe the structure of the bacterial cell with suitable example/ diagram.
f. Write a short note on "Gram's staining technique"

Q 5. Attempt any *four* of the following:

a. What are the factors responsible for cancer causation? What are the measures used in prevention and control of cancer?
b. Describe the causative factors, prevention, care and control of diabetes mellitus.
c. Describe the causative factors, prevention care and control of cardiovascular diseases.
d. Explain various indications of health in short.

e. Describe the different types of immunizing agents with suitable examples.
f. What are hospital acquired infections? How it can be prevented?

Q 6. Give the causative agent, mode of transmission and prevention of any *four* of the following:

a. Leprosy
b. Plague
c. Tuberculosis
d. Polio
e. Rabies
f. Malaria

Winter Examination 2010

D Pharm First Year

Health Education and Community Pharmacy

Q 1. Answer any *five* of the following:

a. Define (any *two*)
   i. Nutrition
   ii. Entomology
   iii. Contraceptives
b. Name a vitamin which causes following deficiency disorder (any *two*)
   i. Beriberi
   ii. Scurvy
   iii. Night blindness
c. Name two airborne infections
d. Give one example of each.
   i. Physical contraceptive methods
   ii. Athropod borne infections
e. Give the long form of (any *two*)
   i. DPT
   ii. HIV
   iii. CHF
f. Draw a flow diagram of rapid sand filter.
g. Name any two fungal infections.

Q 2. Answer any *four* of the following:

a. Enumerate various indicators of health. Describe any one.
b. Write sources, functions and deficiency of vitamin A.
c. Discuss various health determinants.
d. Write a note on 'immunological agents'
e. Give the causative agent, mode of transmission and prevention of tetanus.

Q 3. Answer any *four* of the following:

a. What are vitamins? Classify them.
b. Define communicable diseases. Explain any one surface infection.

c. Name the diseases caused by proteins. Give their symptoms.
d. Define and explain demographic cycle.
e. Write a note on principles of prevention of disease.
f. Explain in detail cardiopulmonary resuscitation.

Q 4. Answer any *four* of the following:

a. What is immunity? Describe any one type of immunity.
b. Define stroke. Give its causes and control.
c. Give the examples of sexually transmitted diseases. Describe any one.
d. Name the causative agent, mode of transmission and control of typhoid.
e. Describe method of isolation of pure culture.
f. Compare Gram +ve and Gram –ve bacteria.

Q 5. Answer any *four* of the following:

a. Define disease. Describe prepathogenesis phase of disease.
b. Draw a well-labelled diagram of bacterial cell.
c. What is family planning? What are the objectives of family planning?
d. What are the health effects of poor light? Name a vitamin synthesized with the help of sunlight.
e. Give the first aid treatment of burns.
f. Describe various method of water purification.

Q 6. Answer any *four* of the following:

a. Discuss type of disinfectants with examples.
b. Give the type of cancer. Enumerate its causes.
c. Describe a permanent method of sterilization for male.
d. Name any one respiratory infection. Give the mode of transmission, prevention and control of it.
e. Define and state the needs of first aid.
f. What are carbohydrates? Give their sources with examples.

Summer Examination 2011

D Pharm First Year

Health Education and Community Pharmacy

Q 1. Answer any *eight* of the following:

a. Define the terms:
   i. Health
   ii. Disease

b. Name the vitamin causing following deficiency disease:
   i. Beriberi
   ii. Scurvy
   iii. Rickets
   iv. Xerophthalmia

c. Write two advantages and two disadvantages of oral contraceptives.

d. Define first aid and list the elements of minor surgery and dressing.

e. Define medical entomology. Name one rodent and disease transmitted by that rodent.

f. Classify microorganisms

g. Write causative agent for (i) Malaria, (ii) Gonorrhoea.

h. What is hypertension? Write prevention and control of hypertension.

i. What do the following acronyms stand for?
   i. BCG
   ii. DPT

j. Define:
   i. Demography
   ii. Family planning

k. Give the composition of balanced diet.

l. Define:
   i. Microbiology
   ii. Virus

Q 2. Answer any *four* of the following:

a. Define the terms:
   i. Physical health
   ii. Mental health
   iii. Social health

b. What is disease agent? Classify them with examples.

c. Classify vitamins and write sources of vitamin A.

d. Name one disease each caused due to deficiency of the following:
   i. Iodine
   ii. Iron
   iii. Vitamin B_{12}
   iv. Fluorine
   v. Folic acid
   vi. Nicotinic acid

e. What first aid treatment should be given in snakebite?

f. Write "Rule of nines" for estimation of percentage of burns. Write emergency treatment for burns.

Q 3. Answer any *four* of the following:

a. Name the different sources of water. State the sources which pollute water.

b. Define noise and state the major ill effects of noise.

c. Define air pollution. What are the major sources of air pollution?

d. With the help of neat labelled diagram, describe the structure of bacteria.

e. Give the method and importance of GEAM staining.

f. Define the terms:
   i. Incubation period
   ii. Epidemiology
   iii. Vaccine

Q 4. Give the causative agent, mode of transmission and prevention of any *four* of the following:

a. Leprosy
b. Tuberculosis
c. Plague
d. AIDS
e. Chickenpox
f. Cholera

Q 5. Answer any *four* of the following:

a. What is diabetes mellitus? Give causes and preventing measures of diabetes mellitus.
b. Discuss the design and mechanism of septic tank.
c. What are Hospital aquired infections? Write prevention and control of nosocomial infections.
d. Give disinfection procedure for
   i. Sputum
   ii. Room
   iii. Dead bodies
e. "Rhythm method for contraception is effective method only for literate couples." Explain the statement with reasons.
f. Give the classification of family planning methods with examples.

Q 6. Answer any *four* of the following:

a. List the various determinants of health and explain any two determinants of health.
b. What is artifical respiration? Explain "Kiss of Life" (mouth to mouth respiration).
c. Give the advantages and disadvantages of condom.
d. What are proteins? Explain sources and deficiency disorders of proteins.
e. Write the types, causative factors and preventative measures of cancer.
f. Define the term immusiation. Write "National Immunisation Schedule".

Winter Examination 2011

D Pharm First Year

Health Education and Community Pharmacy

Q 1. Answer any *five* of the following:

a. Define the term:
   i. Epidemiology
   ii. Demography
b. Name the causative agent for the following diseases:
   i. Tuberculosis
   ii. Diphtheria

c. i. Name one airborne disease
   ii. Name one water bornedisease
d. Enlist the different methods of transmission of diseases.
e. Give the long form of the following abbreviations:
   i. AIDS ii. WHO
   iii. DPT iv. CHD
f. Differentiate between communicable and non-communicable diseases with examples.
g. What is health? Mention various dimensions of health.

Q 2. Answer any *four* of the following:

a. What are the functions and sources of protein?
b. Explain the natural history of diseases.
c. Give the sources and functions of vitamin-C. Explain the symptoms of scurvy.
d. What is cancer? Discuss its prevention and control.
e. What is immunity? Explain active and passive immunity.
f. Explain demographic cycle. Comment on it.

Q 3. Answer any *four* of the following:

a. Explain the diseases caused by proteins with its preventive measures.
b. What are the first aid treatment for snakebite?
c. What are the types of cancer? Explain the factors responsible for cancer.
d. What is family planning? Classify with examples.
e. Give the advantages and disadvantages of oral contraceptives.
f. Give the causative agent, mode of transmission and prevention of malaria.

Q 4. Answer any *four* of the following:

a. What is shock? Describe the first aid treatment for shock.
b. What is balanced diet? What are the common deficiencies in Indian diet?
c. Explain in short the element of minor surgery and dressing.
d. Discuss in detail the concept of disease prevention.
e. Explain different staining techniques for the study of bacteria.
f. Describe various methods of water purification.

Q 5. Answer any *four* of the following:

a. Discuss the role of pharmacist to promote family planning.
b. What is disinfection? Describe in brief various methods of disinfection.

c. What are the causes of Diabetes? How it is prevented?
d. Write a note on Immunization Schedule
e. What is atrifical respiration? Explain mouth to mouth respiration.
f. Name any two diseases transmitted by rodents. Explain how to control rodents.

Q 6. Answer any *four* of the following:

a. What is AIDS? Explain mode of transmission and preventive measures of AIDS.
b. Draw a well labelled diagram of virus. Name any four diseases caused by viruses.
c. Enlist four arthropod borne diseases. Explain in brief different methods of arthropod control.
d. What is hospital acquired infection? Describe mode of transmission and control of hospital acquired infection.
e. What are the composition of pure air? How air pollution can be controlled?
f. Explain in brief the principles of disease control and prevention.

Summer Examination 2012

D Pharm First Year

Health Education and Community Pharmacy

Q 1. Attempt any *eight* of the following:

a. Define the terms:
   i. Mortality   ii. Health
b. Name the vitamin causing following deficiency disease:
   i. Pellagra   ii. Osteomalacia
   iii. Scurvy   iv. Beriberi
c. Write two advantages and two disadvantages of coitus interruptus.
d. Give the first aid treatment for fracture.
e. Name one disease caused by following orthopod:
   i. Housefly   ii. Mosquito
f. Name causative agent of following diseases:
   i. Syphilis   ii. Tuberculosis
g. Name the disease due to following causative agent:
   i. Varicella zoster   ii. *Yersinia pestis*
h. Write prevention and control of diabetes mellitus.
i. What do the following acronyms stand for:
   i. AIDS   ii. TT
   iii. WHO   iv. STD

j. Define:
   i. Contraceptive
   ii. Fertility
k. Give the composition of balanced diet.
l. Classify micro-organisms.

Q 2. Attempt any *four* of the following:

a. Define the terms:
   i. Social health
   ii. Mental health
   iii. Physical health
b. Name various indicators used for measurement of health and explain morbidity indicators.
c. Classify vitamins and write source of vitemin D.
d. What is epidemiology? Discuss its types.
e. Write the emergency treatment given in snakebite.
f. Write "rule of nines" for estimation of percentage of burns. Write first aid treatment for burns.

Q 3. Attempt any *four* of the following:

a. What is air pollution? Mention its causes and prevention.
b. Discuss the design and mechanism of septic tank.
c. Define water pollution. What are the major sources of water pollution?
d. Classify bacteria depending upon their shape.
e. Define staining and explain Gram Staining.
f. Define the terms:
   i. Incubation period
   ii. Disinfection
   iii. Immunity

Q 4. Attempt any *four* of the following:

a. What is hypertension? Give causes and preventive measures of hypertension.
b. Name the methods for small scale purification of water and explain "Boiling method" for purification.
c. What are nosocomial infections? Write prevention and control of nosocomial infections.
d. Give disinfection procedure for:
   i. Faeces and urine
   ii. Sputum
   iii. Instruments
e. Classify family planning methods with examples.
f. Give the three advantages and three disadvantages of condoms.

Q 5. Give the causative agent, mode of transmission and prevention of any *four* of the following diseases:

a. Rabies
b. Diphtheria
c. Typhoid
d. Whooping cough
e. Measles
f. Malaria

Q 6. Attempt any *four* of the following:

a. Explain the concepts of prevention of diseases.
b. What is artifical respiration? Explain "Kiss of life" (mouth to mouth respiration)
c. Give the advantages and disadvantages of intrauterine devices (IUDs)
d. What are vitamins? Explain the sources and deficiency diseases of Vit. A.
e. Write the types, causative factors and preventive measures of cancer.
f. Define the term vaccine. Write "National Immunisation Schedule".

Winter Examination 2012

D Pharm First Year

Health Education and Community Pharmacy

Q 1. Answer any Five of the following:

a. Choose a correct option:
   i. Which of the following is tertiary level of prevention?
      A. Health promotion
      B. Chemoprophylaxis
      C. Rehabilitation
      D. Early diagnosis and treatment
   ii. The body building foods are all except:
      A. Fruits
      B. Milk
      C. Pulses
      D. Poultry
   iii. Third generation IUDs are those which have:
      A. Plastic material
      B. Copper
      C. A hormone
      D. An antispasmodic
   iv. Chickenpox is caused by:
      A. Variola virus
      B. Varicella zoster
      C. Rota virus
      D. Tanapox

b. Define: (any *two*)
   i. Disease
   ii. Health
   iii. Demography

c. Give the long forms of following abbreviations:

i. IDDM	ii. BBT
iii. STD	iv. OPV

d. Name any four arthropods with a disease transmitted by them.
e. What is microbiology? Give its importance.
f. Give one example of each:
   i. Chemical disinfection method
   ii. Waterborne disease
   iii. Source of water supply
   iv. Temporary contraceptive method
g. What is fracture? Name any three types of fractures

Q 2. Answer any *four* of the following:

a. Write in detail the role of a pharmacist in the maintenance of the community health.
b. Discuss in brief hospital acquired infections.
c. Discuss mortality indicators.
d. Write in detail the functions, source of protein and protein energy malnutrition (PEM).
e. Draw a well labelled diagram of bacterial cell. Classify bacteria depending on their oxygen requirement.
f. Give the causes of:
   i. Cancer   ii. Hypertension

Q 3. Answer any *four* of the following:

a. Differentiate between
   i. Vasectomy and tubectomy
   ii. Active and passive immunity
b. Define:
   i. Nutrition
   ii. Medical entomology
   iii. Contraceptive
c. Classify minerals with examples. Explain the role of any one major mineral.
d. Chart out the national immunization schedule.
e. Discuss in detail 'Noise pollution'.
f. Discuss in detail the role of 3rd generation IUDs in national family welfare activities.

Q 4. Answer any *four* of the following:

a. Define and explain demographic cycle.
b. Discuss in detail the first aid treatment provided by a pharmacist to a patient of large area superfacial burns.

c. Describe with a flow diagram "Rapid Stand Filtration method".
d. What is the need for 'Staining'? Describe 'Ziehl-Neelsen method'
e. Describe commonly used antiseptics for dressing.
f. Write a note on 'isolation of pure culture'.

Q 5. Answer any *four* of the following:

a. Give a brief of causes of blindness in India.
b. Enumerate the water soluble vitamins. Give the detail account about the functions, sources and deficiency of vitamin B_{12}.
c. What is water pollution? Give its impact on human life.
d. Write about the purification of water on small scale by chemical disinfection.
e. Justify the statemtne 'Education is the best contraceptives' by giving suitable Indian examples.
f. Define the term "first aid". What are the major principles of first aid treatment?

Q 6. Tabulate the following by giving causative agent, mode of transmission and prevention (any *four*)

a. Measles
b. Typhoid fever
c. Filariasis
d. Trachoma
e. Syphilis
f. Diphtheria

Summer Examination 2013

D Pharm First Year

Health Education and Community Pharmacy

Q 1. Attempt any *eight* of the following:

a. Draw a flow diagram of "Rapid Sand Filtration".
b. Define any *two*:
   i. Entomology
   ii. Essential amino acid
   iii. Epidemiology
c. Name vitamins given in the treatment of following deficiency diseases/disorders.
   i. Bleeding disorder
   ii. Beriberi
   iii. Keratomalacia
   iv. Megaloblastic anemia
d. What do you know about the following?
   i. Reservoir
   ii. Antibody
e. Compare the benign cancer and malignant cancer.

f. Give long form of (any *two*):
   i. IUD
   ii. BCG
   iii. STD
   iv. ORS

g. Define (any *two*):
   i. Immunity
   ii. Infection
   iii. Epidemic

h. State important inorganic elements/minerals related to the following:
   i. Haemoglobin
   ii. Enlargement of thyroids
   iii. Contraction of muscles
   iv. Development of bone

i. Explain in brief (any *one*):
   i. Mortality
   ii. Balance diet

j. Name causative agent of the following:
   i. Measles
   ii. Plague
   iii. Rabies
   iv. Typhoid

k. Explain the term:
   i. Health
   ii. Incubation period

l. Name any two fungal infections.

Q 2. Attempt any *four* of the following:

a. What is fracture? Describe "first aid for fracture".
b. What is sewage? What are aims of sewage treatment?
c. Explain Gram Staining technique.
d. What are nosocomial infection? Describe prevention and control of it.
e. What are effects of air pollution of health? Name two methods of controlling.
f. What are proteins? Explain functions and deficiency diseases of protein.

Q 3. Attempt any *four* of the following:

a. Describe emergency treatment of burns.
b. Describe causes and control of diabetes.
c. Define and explain demographic cycle.
d. Name four dimensions of health and describe physical dimension.
e. What are zoonotic diseases? Give example and controlling measures.
f. Describe the structure of a bacterial cell with a well-labelled diagram.

Q 4. Attempt any *four* of the following:

a. Classify contraceptives with examples.
b. What are carbohydrates? Give sources with examples.
c. Explain sources of water.

d. Give the source and deficiency diseases of vitamin B.
e. Enlist health indicators and explain any two.
f. Explain cardiopulmonary resuscitation.

Q 5. Attempt any *four* of the following:

a. Describe methods of isolation of pure culture.
b. What is natural history of disease? Explain it.
c. What are advantages and disadvantages of light?
d. Describe national immunization schedule.
e. Give prevention and treatment of hypertension.
f. Discuss the "Role of Pharmacist in Community".

Q 6. Give causative agent, mode of transmission and prevention and control of following diseases (any *four*)

a. Polio
b. Leprosy
c. Cholera
d. Trachoma
e. AIDS
f. TB

Winter Examination 2013

D Pharm First Year

Health Education and Community Pharmacy

Q 1. Attempt any *five* of the following:

a. Give causative agent for the following (any *four*):
   i. AIDS
   ii. Plague
   iii. Typhoid
   iv. Chickenpox
   v. Measles

b. State the full form of the following abbreviation:
   i. WHO
   ii. DPT
   iii. BCG
   iv. STD

c. i. Name the disease caused by (any *two*):
   1. *Plasmodium vivax*
   2. *Treponema pallidum*
   3. *Chlamydia trachomatis*

   ii. Define the following terms:
   1. Microbiology
   2. First aid

d. Give one example each for the following (any *four*):
   i. Acid fast bacteria
   ii. Non-communicable disease

iii. Immunizing agent
iv. Chemical disinfectant
v. Permanent method for male sterilization

e. i. Compare communicable and non-communicable diseases, giving examples.
ii. Define the terms 'Incubation Period' and 'Nosocomial Infections'.

f. i. Define the terms 'sterilization' and 'antiseptic'.
ii. Name two airborne and two waterborne diseases.

g. i. Give emergency treatment for snakebite.
ii. Name at least two causative factors for cancer.

Q 2. Attempt any *three* of the following:

a. Define the term 'Health'. Enlist different dimensions of health and explain it.
b. What is 'balanced diet'? Give its expected composition. State the common deficiencies in Indian diet.
c. What is 'family planning'? Classify the methods of family planning with examples.
d. Describe the structure of a bacterial cell with a well labelled diagram.
e. Describe different sources of water supply, giving advantages and disadvantages of each.

Q 3. Attempt any *three* of the following:

a. Discuss the role of a community pharmacist.
b. Define and classify 'Food'.
c. What is 'Cardiopulmonary Resuscitation'? Explain the process of CPR by ABC formula.
d. What are different methods used for purification of water on small scale? Explain.
e. Define the term 'Communicable disease'. Classify different types of communicable diseases with examples.

Q 4. Attempt any *three* of the following:

a. What is 'Demography'? Explain demographic cycle.
b. Define the term 'determinants of health'. Classify them and explain 'Socio-economic conditions' as health determinants.
c. What is meant by PEM? Give its causes and write about Kwashiorkor and marasmus.
d. What are different types of fractures? Discuss first aid treatment for fractures in general.
e. Define 'medical entomology'. Explain different modes of transmission of arthropod borne diseases with examples

Q 5. Attempt any *three* of the following:

a. State the purpose of microbial staining. Explain Gram staining.
b. Name the causatibe agent for tuberculosis. Give its mode of transmission, symptoms and preventive measures to be adopted.
c. What is 'Epidemiology'? Enlist and explain different types of epidemiological methods.
d. Give sources, functions and deficiency manifestations of vitamin A.
e. What is Diabetes Mellitus? Give causative factors, type and measures for prevention-care of diabetes.

Q 6. Attempt any *three* of the following:

a. What is meant by 'Indicators of health'? Enlist and explain different mortality indicators.
b. Define the term 'Fertility'. Explain various factors affecting fertility.
c. How are bacteria classified on the basis of their shape and arrangement?
d. Write the causative agent, symptoms, mode of transmission and prevention of rabies.
e. Define the term 'Immunity'. Give 'National Immunization Schedule.'

Winter Examination 2014

D Pharm First Year

Health Education and Community Pharmacy

Q 1. Answer any *five* of the following:

a. Define the following terms:
   i. Health education
   ii. Community pharmacy
b. Name the vitamin given in the treatment of following disease/disorder:
   i. Bleeding disorders
   ii. Keratomalacia
   iii. Megaloblastic anemia
   iv. Rickets.
c. Define the following terms (any *two*):
   i. Family planning
   ii. Demography
   iii. Contraceptive
d. Define the following terms (any *two*)
   i. Anthropoid-borne diseases
   ii. Incinerator
   iii. Noise

e. Define the term 'Stains'. State the purpose of staining.
f. What are non-communicable diseases? Give three causes of non-communicable diseases.
g. What do you know about?
   i. Epidemology
   ii. 'Case' and 'Carrier'

Q 2. Answer any *four* of the following:

a. Name different aspects of health. Explain any one.
b. Define 'Prevention of disease'. Explain the concepts of prevention of diseases.
c. Define the following terms:
   i. Host
   ii. Agent
   iii. Intervention
   iv. Disease
d. What is cancer? How it is controlled?
e. Discuss types of disinfectants with examples.
f. Write a note on 'Cold chain storage of vaccines'.

Q 3. Answer any *four* of the following:

a. What are proteins? Explain sources and deficiency of proteins.
b. What are sources and functions of vitamin E.
c. What is balanced diet? Give its advantages.
d. Give a brief account of the 'population problem of India'
e. Define fertility. State the factors affecting fertility.
f. Describe any three IUDs used by females for contraception.

Q 4. Answer any *four* of the following:

a. Define 'first aid'. What is its scope and objectives?
b. Define 'Burns'. Explain first aid treatment of burns.
c. Give a brief account of the elements of minor surgery and dressing.
d. Define the following terms:
   i. Microbiology
   ii. Colony
   iii. Mixed culture
   iv. Differential staining
e. Describe general structural features of viruses with the help of a well labelled diagram.
f. Name various methods of isolation of bacteria. Describe in detail any one method.

Q 5. Answer any *four* of the following:

a. Explain the source of water with examples.
b. Explain various steps of 'Slow Sand filtration methods' for water purification.

c. What is solid waste? How is it disposed of?
d. What are the sources of air pollution? Give the effect of air pollution on health.
e. Define 'STD's. Give examples. Discuss prevention of STD's.
f. Classify hormonal contraceptives. Give at least two advantages and two disadvantages of hormonal contraceptives.

Q 6. Tabulate following communicable diseases by giving causative agents, mode of transmission. (Any *seven*)

a. Tuberculosis
b. Diphtheria
c. Chickenpox
d. Gonorrhea
e. Hepatitis A
f. Typhoid fever
g. Malaria
h. Cholera
i. Hookworm infection.

Summer Examination 2015

D Pharm First Year

Health Education and Community Pharmacy

Q 1. Attempt any *eight* of the following:

a. Name the vitamin causing the following deficiency diseases:
   i. Rickets
   ii. Night blindness
   iii. Scurvy
   iv. Pellagra
b. Define the terms:
   i. Disease
   ii. Health
c. Write the role of pharmacist in promoting family welfare/planning.
d. Name the orthropod transmitting following diseases:
   i. Plague
   ii. Kala-azar
   iii. Cholera
   iv. Malaria
e. Give the emergency treatment for shock.

f. Name causative agent of the following diseases:
   i. Rabies
   ii. Chickenpox
g. Name the disease due to the following causative agent:
   i. *Treponema pallidum*
   ii. *Bordetella pertussis*
h. Write prevention and control of coronary heart diseases.
i. What do the following acronyms stand for?
   i. HIV
   ii. TT
   iii. RNA
   iv. STD
j. What is balanced diet?
k. Define fertility and name the four factors affecting fertility.
l. Draw well-labelled diagram of bacteria cell.

Q 2. Attempt any *four* of the following:

a. Name various indicators used for measurement of health and explain mortality indicators.
b. Define the terms:
   i. Physical health
   ii. Social health
   iii. Mental health
c. Define immunity. Discuss its types.
d. Classify vitamins and write sources of vitamin C.
e. Write the elements of minor surgery and dressing.

Q 3. Attempt any *four* of the following:

a. Classify bacteria depending upon their shape.
b. Define staining and explain acid-fast staining.
c. Define noise and state ill-effects of noise.
d. Discuss the design and mechanism of septic tank.
e. What are the major sources of water pollution? How water pollution can be prevented?
f. Define the terms:
   i. Incubation period
   ii. Epidemiology
   iii. Antiseptic

Q 4. Attempt any *four* of the following:

a. Write causes and preventive measures of cancer.
b. Classify family planning methods with examples.

c. Give three advantages and three disadvantages of oral contraceptives.
d. Name the methods for large scale purification of water and explain "slow sand filtration" for purification.
e. What are hospital acquired infections? Write prevention and control of hospital acquired infections.
f. Write disinfection procedure for:
   i. Dead bodies
   ii. Faeces and urine
   iii. Room

Q 5. Give the causative agent, mode of transmission and prevention of any *four* of the following diseases:

a. Leprosy
b. AIDS
c. Cholera
d. Tuberculosis
e. Influenza
f. Plague

Q 6. Attempt any *four* of the following:

a. Explain "Natural history of disease".
b. Give the advantages and disadvantages of condoms.
c. Write sources and deficiency diseases of vitamin B_1 and vitamin B_{12}.
d. Define the term vaccine. Write "National Immunisation Schedule".
e. What is artificial respiration? Explain "Kiss of Life" (mouth to mouth respiration).
f. Write causative factors, prevention, care and control of diabetes mellitus.

Winter Examination 2015

D Pharm First Year

Health Education and Community Pharmacy

Q 1. Answer any *eight* of the following:

a. Define the terms:
   i. Disease
   ii. Spiritual health
b. Name the vitamin causing following deficiency disease:
   i. Rickets
   ii. Night blindness

iii. Pellagra
iv. Beriberi

c. Write two advantages and two disadvantages of vasectomy for family planning.
d. Explain "kiss of life" for artificial respiration.
e. Name two arthropod-borne diseases and two air-borne diseases.
f. Classify micro-organisms.
g. Write mode of transmission for tuberculosis.
h. How hypertension can be prevented and controlled?
i. What do the following acronyms stand for?
   i. TT
   ii. BCG
   iii. DPT
   iv. AIDS
j. Give two advantages and two disadvantages of intrauterine devices.
k. Name one disease each caused due to deficiency of the following:
   i. Calcium
   ii. Iodine
   iii. Iron
   iv. Folic acid
l. Classify bacteria depending upon their shape.

Q 2. Answer any *four* of the following:

a. List the various determinants of health and explain any one.
b. Define the terms:
   i. Physical health
   ii. Mental health
   iii. Social health
c. Write the composition of balanced diet.
d. Classify vitamins and write sources, deficiency symptoms of Riboflavin (vitamin B_2)
e. Write "Rule of Nines" for estimation of percentage of burns. Write emergency treatment for burns.
f. Name types of fractures and write first aid treatment for fracture.

Q 3. Answer any *four* of the following:

a. Name the methods for solid waste disposal and explain any one.
b. State the major ill effects of noise and dim light.
c. Define water pollution. How water pollution can be prevented and controlled?
d. Give the method and importance of GRAM staining.
e. With the help of neat labelled diagram, describe the structure of bacteria.

f. Give disinfection procedure for:
   i. Dead bodies
   ii. Linen
   iii. Urine

Q 4. Answer any *four* of the following:

a. What is hypertension? Give causes and preventive measures of diabetes mellitus.
b. Discuss the slow sand filter for purification of water.
c. What are hospital acquired infections? Write prevention and control of nosocomial infections.
d. Define the terms:
   i. Epidemiology
   ii. Immunity
   iii. Incubation period
e. Define demography and explain population problem in India.
f. Define fertility and name the factors affecting fertility.

Q 5. Give the causative agent, mode of transmission and prevention of any *four* of the following:

a. Influenza
b. Cholera
c. Leprosy
d. Gonorrhea
e. Whooping cough
f. Plague

Q 6. Answer any *four* of the following:

a. What is disease agent? Classify them.
b. Define first aid and write first aid treatment for snake bite.
c. Write the classification of family planning methods with examples.
d. Classify food and write functions of carbohydrates and proteins.
e. Write the types, causative factors and preventive measures of cancer.
f. Define the term "Immunisation". Write "National Immunisation Schedule".

Summer Examination 2016

D Pharm First Year

Health Education and Community Pharmacy

Q 1. Answer any *eight* of the following:

a. Define the terms:
   i. Balanced diet
   ii. Medical entomology

b. Name a deficiency disease of the following nutrients:
   i. Vitamin D
   ii. Vitamin B_1
   iii. Iodine
   iv. Protein

c. Define the terms:
   i. Nutrition
   ii. Disinfection

d. Give long forms of the following abbreviations:
   i. BCG
   ii. MMR
   iii. TT
   iv. WHO

e. Give two examples each of the following
   i. Physical methods of contraception
   ii. Acid-fast bacteria

f. What do you know about
   i. Concurrent disinfection
   ii. Terminal disinfection

g. Define the terms:
   i. Diabetes mellitus
   ii. Microbiology

h. Name different sources of water.

i. Enumerate various indicators of health.

j. Write causes of air pollution.

k. Write mode of transmission of:
   i. Rabies
   ii. Tetanus

1. Classify immunising agents.

Q 2. Answer any *four* of the following:

a. Write sources, functions, deficiency diseases of vitamin A.

b. Define the term demography. Explain demographic cycle.

c. Enumerate determinants of health. Explain any one.

d. Define nosocomial infections. Write prevention and control of nosocomial infections.

e. Write first aid for shock.

f. Write importance and procedure of 'gram staining'.

Q 3. Answer any *four* of the following:

a. Define blindness. Write causes, prevention and control of blindness.

b. Enlist different methods of isolation of bacteria. Explain any one.

c. Write about hormonal contraceptives.
d. Describe various methods of small scale purification of water.
e. Write first aid treatment for snake bite.
f. Discuss in detail noise pollution.

Q 4. Answer any *four* of the following:

a. Define hypertension. Write causes, prevention and control of hypertension.
b. Explain natural history of disease and its phases.
c. Name various methods of solid waste disposal. Explain any one.
d. Describe structure of virus with the help of a labelled diagram.
e. Give disinfection procedure for
   i. Faeces and urine
   ii. Sputum
f. Explain back pressure arm lift method.

Q 5. Answer any *four* of the following:

Write causative agent, symptoms, prevention and control of

a. Tuberculosis
b. Poliomyelitis
c. Hepatitis
d. Malaria
e. Trachoma
f. AIDS

Q 6. Answer any *four* of the following:

a. Define fertility. Write about various factors which affect fertility.
b. Explain the terms:
   i. Physical health
   ii. Social health
c. Define cancer. Write causes, prevention and control of cancer.
d. Define immunisation. Write about National Immunisation Schedule.
e. Write functions and deficiency disease of:
   i. Iron
   ii. Calcium
f. Define fracture. Name types of fracture and first aid treatment for fracture.

Winter Examination 2016

D Pharm First Year

Health Education and Community Pharmacy

Q 1. Solve any *eight* of the following:

a. Define the terms:
   i. Health education
   ii. Communicable disease
b. Name the disease caused by (any two)
   i. Varicella zoster
   ii. *Bordetella pertussis*
   iii. *Plasmodium vivax*
c. Write scope of first aid.
d. State the full form of the following abbreviations:
   i. HIV
   ii. TT
   iii. BCG
   iv. DPT
e. Write the role of pharmacist in family planning.
f. Write sources and deficiency disease of vitamin A.
g. Define:
   i. Epidemiology
   ii. Incubation period
h. Write composition of balanced diet.
i. Name the vitamin causing the following deficiency disease:
   i. Beriberi
   ii. Pellagra
   iii. Rickets
   iv. Scurvy
j. Write immunization schedule for children.
k. Draw well-labelled diagram of bacterial cell.
l. Differentiate between natural immunity and artificial immunity.

Q 2. Solve any *four* of the following:

a. Write any six indicators of health.
b. Enlist different types of fractures. Write general first aid treatment for fractures.
c. Write sources, functions and deficiency diseases of thiamine (vitamin B_1).
d. Name water-borne diseases. Write about slow sand filter.
e. Discuss demographic cycle.
f. Discuss methods of solid-waste disposal.

Q 3. Solve any *four* of the following:

a. Write note on Gram staining method.
b. Write note on food poisoning.
c. Define medical entomology. Write note on insect control.
d. Write causes, transmission and control of tuberculosis.
e. What are sources of air pollution? Write its effect on health.
f. Write symptoms and first-aid treatment for shock.

Q 4. Solve any *four* of the following:

a. Write notes on noise pollution.
b. Write about types and prevention and control of diabetes mellitus.
c. Differentiate between case control study and cohort study of epidemiology.
d. Classify contraceptive methods with examples.
e. Discuss sources of deficiency diseases due to proteins.
f. Discuss cardio-pulmonary resuscitation (CPR).

Q 5. Solve any *four* of the following:

a. Write about deficiency diseases due to iron and iodine.
b. Write about hormonal contraceptives.
c. Write disinfection procedure for
    i. Room
    ii. Sputum
d. Write natural history of disease with its phases.
e. Write causes, prevention and control of cancer.
f. Discuss in brief about Nosocomial infections.

Q 6. Write causative agent, mode of transmission symptoms and control of the following: (Any four)

a. Typhoid Fever
b. Filariasis
c. Syphilis
d. Leprosy
e. Trachoma
f. Cholera

Summer Examination 2017

D Pharm First Year

Health Education and Community Pharmacy

Q 1. Answer any *eight* of the following:

a. Define Health Education.
b. Enlist any 4 indicators of health.

c. State the functions of fats.
d. Enlist water soluble vitamins.
e. Define the term demography and fertility.
f. Classify the hormonal contraceptives.
g. Enlist the contents of "First Aid Kit".
h. Define the term Microbiology.
i. Enlist any 4 communicable diseases.
j. What are the characteristics of cancer?
k. Define immunity.
l. Define antiseptics with 2 examples.

Q 2. Answer any *four* of the following:

a. Give an account of determinants of Health.
b. Write classifications of food.
c. Write note on cold chain storage of vaccines.
d. Write in detail different stages of demographic cycle.
e. Enlist the methods of contraceptives with examples.
f. Write the emergency treatment of shock.

Q 3. Answer any *four* of the following:

a. Describe the Resuscitation method in detail.
b. Write different sources of water.
c. Define Health. Write the effect of Air pollution on Health.
d. Discuss the purification of water on small scale.
e. Draw the labelled diagram of bacterial cell.
f. Write note on types of fungi and fungal infections.

Q 4. Answer any *four* of the following:

a. Write the life cycle of malarial parasite.
b. Define diabetes mellitus (DM). Write the signs and symptoms of DM.
c. Enumerate the risk factors and prevention of coronary heart diseases.
d. Discuss modes of transmission of diseases.
e. Define Epidemiology and discuss major components of epidemiology.
f. What is disinfection? Describe various methods of disinfection.

Q 5. Answer any *four* of the following:

a. Discuss Hospital Acquired Infections.
b. Write the advantages and disadvantages of condom.
c. Write the first aid treatment for snake bite.
d. Discuss methods of solid waste disposal.

e. Enlist staining techniques for bacteria and explain any one.
f. Write a note on Immunisation Schedule.

Q 6. Write about causative agent, mode of transmission, symptoms and prevention for following infections (any 4):

a. Rabies
b. Filariasis
c. Tuberculosis
d. Leprosy
e. Typhoid fever
f. Chickenpox
g. Cholera